POCKET
HERBAL
REFERENCE
GUIDE

DEBRA ST. CLAIRE

The Crossing Press • Freedom, CA

Pocket Guides from The Crossing Press

Pocket Guide to Acupressure Points for Women
By Cathryn Bauer
$6.95 • Paper • ISBN 0-89594-879-6

Pocket Guide to Fortunetelling
By Scott Cunningham
$6.95 • Paper • ISBN 0-89594-875-3

Pocket Macrobiotics
By Carl Ferre
$6.95 • Paper • ISBN 0-89594-848-6

Pocket Guide to Meditation
By Alan Pritz
$6.95 • Paper • ISBN 0-89594-886-9

Pocket Guide to Visualization
By Helen Graham
$6.95 • Paper • ISBN 0-89594-885-0

Pocket Guide to Bach Flower Essences
By Rachelle Hasnas
$6.95 • Paper • ISBN 0-89594-865-6

Pocket Guide to Naturopathic Medicine
By Judith Boice
$6.95 • Paper • ISBN 0-89594-821-4

Please look for these books at your local bookstore or order from
The Crossing Press, P.O. Box 1048, Freedom, CA 95019.
Add $2.50 for the first book and 50¢ for each additional book.
Or call toll-free 800-777-1048 with your credit card order.

CONTENTS

Introduction

In order to use this herbal guide wisely, it is essential that you understand some basic principles of herbology. Hippocrates stated, "Let your food be your medicine and your medicine be your food." Most of the food plants that we currently use have medicinal properties. For instance, Celery and Parsley have diuretic effects; Apples, Prunes and the Squash family have laxative effects; certain spices such as Black Pepper and Ginger have stimulant effects; etc.

The use of plants as medicines is our oldest form of healing, and traditional botanically based medicine is still the predominant form of medical treatment in today's world. At certain periods in human history, herbalism had peaks of knowledge and usage, the last one being in the late 1800's during the reign of the eclectic physicians. After the ability to synthesize medicine from inert substances such as petroleum and minerals was developed, the therapeutic use of herbs diminished. The art of pharmacy turned to the production of drugs which could bring the quickest relief of symptoms, ignoring the reason that the symptoms appeared.

As we look back, perhaps it is time to reconsider that path. The use of these substances has spawned a myriad of unexpected problems, such as suppression of the very signals that our bodies produce to alert us to a need for change. Pain itself is a call to action—a call to remedy an imbalance in our life-style. From the perspective of Ayurvedic medicine (the oldest recorded healing system), the period of body imbalance which is easiest to correct is that first, often vague sense of unrest which precedes the onset of an illness. The proficient use of herbal therapy is directly connected to our ability to sense that first signal and to adjust our lifestyles accordingly. It is when these signals are continually ignored that disease has a chance to seat itself more deeply within our bodies.

The appropriate use of herbs is only one of many healthy alternatives to our present medical system. It is my hope that as you use this booklet, you will be inspired to explore your own lifestyle and body balance and to study this and other forms of natural healing as you take increasing responsibility for your own health.

Our government is faced with an incredible resurgence of interest in natural healing. While creating laws which were originally designed to protect people from medical fraud, it unfortunately included laws which limit our freedom to choose our own form of medical treatment. Herbs are currently tossed back and forth between "food" and "drug" classifications like a hot potato with no place to rest. With due respect for traditional cultures, and the thousands of years of clinical experience which they represent, herbalists propose that a third classification be created for medicinal plants, namely as agents of traditional medicine, with proven safety being the criteria instead of medical efficacy. Once out of the realm of food and drug, more responsibility would lie with the consumer as to personal use.

Because of the often well-founded prohibition on practicing medicine without a license, making medical claims, etc., the research presented in this booklet must be used only as a guide to the historical use of herbs. Each person's body chemistry is different, and what works for one may not work for another. Your personal responsibility is to pay attention to your own body's reaction to the herbs, and to adjust your use of them as necessary.

I believe that as people turn to natural plant-based medicine, they will rediscover their appreciation for the earth. Due to the increase of industrialization and its destructive effect on the environment, we are losing one species of plants each day, and it is estimated that if the current pattern prevails, it could soon be one species per hour. Once a genetic code is lost, it can never be regained. We are losing potential foods and medicines which could be the solutions to our most important health issues.

As herbalists, we believe that ecological stewardship is essential; therefore, we are faced with several issues as we produce our herbal products. As the use of herbal medicine increases, we could easily extinguish our stands of wild herbs; thus our goal is to protect all plant species and to organically grow the plants we use so that we can insure their survival and continued availability on our planet.

A final note: For goodness sake be sensible about all this…if symptoms persist, pay attention to them. It is always advantageous to seek the diagnostic services of a qualified wholistic physician. If you experience nausea or any other adverse reaction, stop taking the herbs! Too many people, familiar with the terms "detoxification" and "healing crisis," put up with unpleasant reactions to natural products in the belief that these reactions are part of the process of healing (penance for past improprieties?), when, in fact, the body is communicating its need for an adjustment in the choice of therapy. Your skill at interpreting your own body's language will improve with practice; in the meantime, when in doubt, stop what you're doing and study! There is a list of some of the most useful herbal and natural therapy texts at the end of this booklet. *Use them.*

Frequently Asked Questions About Herbal Medicine

I hear the word "herb" pronounced two different ways. Which is correct?

In every country in the world except the United States, the word is pronounced *with* the "h," as in "house." Therefore, many people are ceasing to pronounce it as "erb."

What is a herbal extract?

Herbal extracts are the medicinal properties of herbs extracted into fluids which act as solvents and preservatives such as grain alcohol/distilled water, vinegar or glycerin. No heat is needed in the extraction, therefore the volatile oils and healing properties are preserved.

How do herbal extracts work?

Herbal extracts support the body's ability to heal itself by cleansing and strengthening the tissues. They also catalyze certain body actions, such as diuresis (urination) or diaphoresis (sweating). Extracts are quickly assimilated by the body, and are best used to support and maintain the body's own efforts to defend itself from disease. Therefore herbal extracts play an important role in preventive medicine.

Why take a herbal extract instead of other forms of herbal preparations?

Extracts are the most convenient way to ingest herbal medicines. Capsules and most teas are made from dried herbs, and their potency is vulnerable. Herbal extracts can be produced from *fresh* plants, and maintain their potency for 3-5 years if stored out of direct sunlight in a cool place. They do not require refrigeration.

How are herbal extracts taken?

Many people prefer diluting the dosage (usually 20-30 drops) with 1/2 cup water, then drinking it like an instant "tea." If there is an acute problem like a sore throat, however, it can be squirted back so that it coats the throat full strength. Hold the dropper forward so that it doesn't touch the mouth to preserve its sterility.

Is it necessary to use alcohol in herbal extracts?

Yes. The medicinal constituents of plants fall into two basic categories—water soluble and alcohol soluble. Many constituents are not water soluble and will only give up their medicinal properties to an alcohol base. If only water is used, the alcohol soluble constituents will remain in the plant matter and not be bio-available. Therefore, a specific balance of distilled water and grain alcohol is required to extract the full spectrum of medicinal properties from the plant.

What if one does not want the alcohol?

If you want to remove the alcohol, put the dose in a cup, pour 1/2 cup hot water over it, and let it sit, uncovered, for 5 minutes. The alcohol will dissipate, leaving the herbal concentrate behind. (The amount of alcohol in an average dose [30 drops] of a herbal extract containing 50% alcohol is roughly equivalent to 1/50 of a can of beer.)

What is the proper amount to take?

Always a sticky subject due to personal metabolism, dietary habits, stress levels and other vagaries of our individual bodies, dosage guidelines are nevertheless important. Well put in Felter's *Materia Medica*, Vol. 1, "It is better to err on the side of insufficient dosage and trust to nature, than to overdose to the present or future harm or danger to the patient." In other words, try a little, and watch for your reaction, before you take a lot. In acute cases people have taken a dropperful every hour and usually take 1-3 droppers full per day in chronic problems. If one is sensitive enough, and listens well to one's own body, the dosage should be apparent. If you have dosage questions, consult a competent wholistic practitioner for assistance.

Can herbs be taken with prescription drugs?

The key is to use herbs and a healthy diet to correct the imbalance before prescription drugs are necessary. Consult a wholistic physician with botanical training for the herb's compatibility with specific prescriptions.

What is the difference between Chinese, Ayurvedic and American herbal products?

Other than the locality of their production, the real difference between the three is in the diagnostic systems which are the foundation of their use. The plant itself is no more efficient just because it was grown in another country.

American herbal products are often associated with the western medical model, which treats symptoms instead of the cause of the "dis-ease." The Chinese and Ayurvedic systems use herbs as *foods* to increase the body's systemic integrity. American herbs can be used in the same manner.

U.S. regulations require spraying of imported plant products which are not pre-packaged. These fumigants and other chemicals leave a residue on the plants which I feel make them unsuitable for medicinal purposes. It is also difficult to guarantee whether the plants were organically grown or fumigated prior to packaging.

When we utilize locally grown U.S. plants, we can closely monitor their growing and harvesting conditions to assure the highest standards of quality, while also supporting the local economy.

Why do some manufacturers use fresh herbs in their extracts instead of dried ones?

Because they feel that the best extract is made by capturing the *vital potency* of the *fresh plant*. The greater the distance and time between harvest and processing, the greater chance of quality deterioration in the final product. Dried plants are exposed to the influences of moisture, atmosphere and in-storage contamination. From the time they are gathered until they are used, a constant change is occurring. Oxidation, the loss of volatile oils, and other biochemical breakdowns decrease the quality of the product. Fresh plants are also much easier to identify, thus preventing the substitution of inferior materials.

The Language of Herbal Preparation & Usage

The array of teas, capsules, extracts and tinctures displayed on the market shelves can be confusing. Questions like "what is the difference between an extract and a tincture?" are often heard. The following section provides insight into the basic language of herbology. Once you have become acquainted with the fundamental terminology, understanding how and when to use the various preparations will easily follow.

FLUID PREPARATIONS

The chemical constituents found in plant life dissolve in different types of fluids. The following list is organized according to solvency.

Water Based Preparations

Infusion

Extraction of the medicinal or flavor elements of plants by soaking in cold or hot water. Used for leaves, stems and flowers.

Decoction

Extraction of medicinal constituents by gently simmering the denser parts of plants for extended periods of time. (i.e. roots, barks, seeds, etc.)

Medicinal or Beverage Tea

Prepared by placing the herbs in a vessel of water (preferably distilled) which has just been boiled, then stirring, covering and letting steep for 10-15 min. (Can also be made as a cold infusion.)

Hydro-Alcoholic Preparations

These preparations are best made with a mixture of distilled water and pure grain alcohol (ETOH).

> *Weight/volume ratio refers to the proportion of **plant** to the **liquid** it is being extracted into: i.e. water, grain alcohol, vinegar, etc. More plant matter does not necessarily increase the potency of the extract, as the point is to adequately "saturate" the plant matter in order to extract the full spectrum of available constituents (impossible if there is not enough liquid to "flush" out the active ingredients).*

USP Fluid Extract

- **Weight/volume ratio:** 1:1 (Herb weight & liquid volume are equal, producing an extract in which 1 cc =1 gm dried herb.)
- **Extraction method:** Percolation of dried plant material according to specifications in United States or British Pharmacoepias.
- **Quality control:** It is harder to identify adulterations of dried and pulverized specimens without chemical analysis. Imported herbs and those in storage are subjected to chemical sprays to prevent insect infestation and molds.
- **Note:** The advantage of drying a plant is that it concentrates some medicinal properties. Unfortunately, important constituents are lost along the way. This is particularly evident in botanicals which have been pulverized and undergo long periods of storage before extraction, leading to oxidation and rancidity.

Fresh Plant Fluid Extract

- **Weight/volume ratio:** By the time reliable research on *fresh* plant extraction had begun, the focus of pharmacy had shifted to isolation and synthesis of active constituents. Therefore, fresh plant or "green extractions" had limited reference in the early pharmacoepias. As a result, there is a lack of standardized definition in the industry. We are only now, in the recent rise of interest in botanical medicine, able to redefine and perfect this processing technique. Most manufacturers define them as highly concentrated extracts prepared in a range between 1:0.75 and 1:3, depending on moisture analysis and the physical nature of the fresh plant.
- **Extraction method:** Maceration (Grinding up and blending with dissolving solution for specified period)
- **Quality control:** Plants should be set into the menstruum (the combination of plant matter and dissolving fluid) as soon as possible after harvesting, optimum being no later than 24 hours. All plants should be organically grown or ecologically wildcrafted in pure surroundings, away from power lines or environmental pollutants.
- **Note:** Most botanicals can and should be extracted while fresh. A few are dried to alter potentially irritating constituents, as in the case of Cascara Sagrada.

Tincture

- **Weight/volume ratio:** 1:5
- **Extraction method:** Maceration (fresh or dried plants) or percolation (dried plants)
- **Quality control:** Process techniques vary. Question manufacturer about plant condition at time of extraction (fresh or dry, length of time between harvest and extraction). Ask about extraction method.
- **Notes:** Less strong than the first two categories. Can be prepared with either fresh or dried plants, depending on

method of extraction, although standard definition of tincture indicates the use of dried material.

Homeopathic Mother Tincture

- **Weight/volume ratio:** 1:10
- **Extraction method:** Maceration, most often prepared with fresh plants.
- **Quality control:** As above
- **Notes:** Generally used as a base for further dilutions and sucussions as per standard homeopathic pharmacy technique.

Solid Extract

- **Weight/volume ratio:** Generally 4:1
- **Extraction method:** 1) With fresh plants, maceration then concentration from a liquid down into a solid, utilizing the rotary evaporation technique. 2) Dried plants are usually percolated, then concentrated.
- **Quality control:** As above. Ask manufacturer if extraction is performed in line with advertised quality standards or performed as an out-lab service.

Elixirs

"Elixirs are sweetened, aromatic and spiritous solutions, designed as vehicles for small amounts of active medicines. As a class they are very unsatisfactory, though pleasant preparations."
—*The Eclectic Materia Medica*, Pharmacology and Therapeutics, H.W. Felter, MD

Essential Oils

The pure, volatile, aromatic essence of the plant. Usually steam distilled, although there are other methods such as effleurage and direct expression.

Glycerites

Vegetable Glycerin is a hydrolized vegetable fat which is between water and alcohol in its ability to dissolve plant constituents. It has weaker preservative properties than alcohol. Very sweet taste, making it useful in the preparation of elixirs and syrups. Glycerites are most safely made with dried herbs to prevent spoilage, because fresh plants have higher percentages of active bacteria.

Herbal Oils

Created by soaking or gently simmering herbs in a carrier oil such as olive or almond.

Syrups

Syrups are generally made by simmering fresh or dried herbs down into a concentrate. Honey, glycerin, Sucanat, Nutri-Cane, maple syrup, rice syrup or other natural sweeteners are added, then simmered down until the mixture reaches the desired syrupy consistency. Quick syrups can also be made by adding herbal extracts to honey or other sweeteners, with the advantage of not using heat. This method best preserves the volatile constituents.

Vinegars

Vinegar also dissolves medicinal constituents, however, it is not as effective as the hydro-alcoholic solution. Its preservative strength is more than plain water and less than alcohol. Will extract constituents from fresh or dried herbs.

DRIED HERBS

Herbs are also available in dry form. They should be purchased from companies who utilize organically grown herbs. Smell them to see if the aromas are still present, one indication of proper harvesting and storage. Store in tightly closed glass containers away from direct sunlight. If properly cared for, their potency lasts approximately one year.

Bulk Herbs

May be used to brew beverage or medicinal teas, make poultices, baths, steams and a number of other herbal preparations. Available in single herbs or combinations.

Tea Bags

Should be purchased in bleach free paper to avoid dioxin contamination. A very easy way to prepare herbal beverages. Also useful as emergency poultices.

Capsulated Herbs

As of this printing, the new animal free gelatin capsules still have some problems with early disintegration, which are expected to be corrected soon. The problem with gelatin capsules is that they short circuit the digestive process by prohibiting oral "recognition" of the herb. I have seen many cases where they moved through the entire digestive tract and were eliminated as a whole capsule without ever opening. Although it may not taste good, it helps to open one capsule and sprinkle it over the rest of the capsules in the jar. This way the body has a greater chance of secreting the proper digestive enzymes by analyzing the "taste"—similar to the social courtesy of telephoning before you visit.

Another issue is the difficulty in swallowing capsules. They should not be given to small children. Open the capsule and mix it with a carrier such as a bit of honey. (This type of herbal preparation is known as an electuary.)

Powders

When a herb is broken down in small enough particles to be considered a powder, it has a much shorter shelf life, due to the fact that more surface area is exposed to oxygen and light. The volatile oils and other medicinal constituents are easily lost, decreasing the potency.

Herbs are powdered previous to the capsulation process and in the percolation process of using dried herbs to make fluid extracts. Some companies also provide them as powdered formulas.

If you must use powdered herbs, it is best to powder them immediately before use. This is most easily accomplished with a coffee grinder or mortar and pestle.

GLOSSARY OF
HERBAL PREPARATIONS

Balm: See *Salve*

Baths: Water based infusion designed to achieve herbal therapy through immersion/osmosis.

Capsules: Inclusion of dried, powdered herbs in gelatin, primarily to hide their taste.

Cerates: A fatty preparation resembling an ointment, but having a firmer consistency and a higher melting point. True cerates always contain wax.

Cold Compresses: Used to prevent swelling and reduce fevers. An infusion or decoction which is chilled, soaked into a cloth and externally applied.

Creams: Herbs captured in a fatty or oily base with a light, airy texture which is easily spread on skin for a healing or moisturizing effect.

Decoctions: Roots, barks, seeds and other dense plant parts gently simmered for extended periods to dissolve water soluble constituents.

Douches: An infusion or decoction administered vaginally to cleanse, disinfect and soothe.

Electuaries: The medicinal or nourishing constituents of herbs in a sweet base such as honey.

Elixirs: Thin, syrupy liquid carrier used to make herbs more palatable. Very sweet.

Enemas: Infusion or decoction rectally injected to relieve constipation, cleanse and soothe the large intestine.

Eyewashes: Infusion or decoction used to cleanse, disinfect and soothe ocular tissue.

Fluid Extracts: The medicinal properties of herbs in a concentrated liquid form for internal consumption or external application.

Fomentation: Applied hot—an infusion or decoction of herbs soaked into a cloth for external application.

Gargle: An infusion, decoction or diluted extract used to cleanse, disinfect and soothe the throat. Normally not swallowed.

Glycerites: The medicinal or nourishing constituents of herbs extracted into this highly sweet hydrolized vegetable fat. Does not sufficiently extract full spectrum of available constituents.

Granules: Sugar pellets impregnated with medicinal matter which is applied in liquid form and absorbed by the pellets, then dried. Usually used as a carrier for homeopathic preparations.

Infusions: Leaves, flowers and other tender parts of plants soaked in freshly boiled water to capture their water soluble constituents. Internal and external use.

Juices: See *Succus*

Liniments: Alcoholic or hydro-alcoholic solutions of medicinal constituents used for external application.

Lotions: Oil/water based preparation, allowing healing benefits to be absorbed through skin.

Lozenges: Small, sweetened, candy-like disks or drops (preferably with natural base ingredients) which are sucked to obtain medicinal benefit (dependent on specific formula).

Mucilages: Fresh or dried herbs which become slick and slimy when mixed with water. Used internally and externally to soothe and heal irritated tissue.

Ointments: Herbs mixed with lard, lanolin, petroleum or wax for external application to skin afflictions. Gradually melts with skin heat and is absorbed.

Oxymel: Neutralizes acrid or pungent taste of herbs like Garlic with vinegar and honey.

Pessaries: Bullet sized, cocoa butter based pellet which carries herbs for vaginal absorption.

Pills: Masses of medicinal matter, round or oval in shape, designed for internal consumption. Sometimes contain carrier material such as starch, gelatin or milk sugar.

Plasters: Medicinal herbs stirred into a sticky base which is then spread on skin, silk, cotton cloth or paper. Solidifies into a hard mass which mechanically supports the injured area while the medicinal constituents are absorbed.

Poultices: Fresh or dried herbs mixed with enough liquid to make a thick, pasty consistency for external application to skin and muscular injuries.

Powders: Dried herbs comminuted (ground) into small particles for encapsulation or extraction.

Salves: Oil and beeswax preparation useful for external skin application to promote healing of injured skin. Also known as a *Balm*.

Sinus Snuff: A powdered herb mixture designed for nasal inhalation. Produces copious discharge, aiding decongestion of the sinuses.

Spray: Herbal extracts, teas or diluted essential oils in spray bottles for internal or external use.

Steams: Infusion or decoction of herbs or small amounts of essential oils in hot water which rises up and surrounds the affected area for a detoxifying or decongesting effect.

Succus: Freshly expressed herbal juice, usually preserved with grain alcohol.

Suppositories: Bullet shaped pellets of powdered herbs in a cocoa butter base designed for rectal absorption.

Syrups: Sweet, thick carrier for herbal medicine. Base usually consists of honey, glycerin, maple syrup, rice syrup, etc.

Tablets: Dry or moistened powdered herbs compressed into a variety of swallowable shapes. Sometimes contain carrier material such as starch, gelatin or milk sugar.

Tinctures: Herbal constituents extracted into a standard weight/volume ratio of 1 part herb to 5 parts solvent.

Vinegars: Herbal constituents dissolved into vinegar for internal ingestion. Should be raw apple cider vinegar.

Wines: Herbal constituents dissolved into wines. Adds flavor. Best made with organic wines.

THERAPEUTIC ACTIONS

Abortifacient: Produces abortion

Adaptogenic: Decreases the harmful effects of stress

Alterative: Promotes healthy changes in the organism

Analgesic: Relieves pain

Anaphrodisiac: Subdues sexual desire

Anesthetic: Produces insensibility to pain

Anodyne: Relieves pain

Antacid: Counteracts acidity

Antagonist: Opposes action of other medicines

Antidote: Counteracts effect of poison

Antiemetic: Prevents vomiting

Antigalactic: Diminishes secretion of milk

Anthelmintic: Destroys parasites

Antihypnotic: Prevents sleep

Anti-inflammatory: Reduces inflammation

Antilithic: Helps prevent stone or gravel

Antimicrobial: Destroys microbes

Antimycetic: Destroys fungal infections

Antiseptic: Prevents or arrests putrefaction

Antispasmodic: Reduces spasms, relaxes

Antitussive: Relieves or prevents coughs

Aperient: Gently laxative

Aphrodisiac: Stimulates sexual desire

Astringent: Contracts tissue, restrains discharges

Bactericide: Destroys bacteria

Bitter: Increases tone and activity of gastric mucosa

Calmative: Gently calms nerves

Cardiac: Heart stimulant or tonic

Carminative: Prevents or relieves flatulence

Cathartic: Hastens or increases evacuation of the bowels

Cholagogue: Stimulates flow of bile

Demulcent: Soothing to mucus membranes

Deodorant: Removes/corrects foul odors

Depuritive: Removes impurities from the body, cleansing action

Diaphoretic: Increases perspiration

Digestant: Aids digestion

Disinfectant: Destroys the cause of infection

Diuretic: Increases secretion of urine

Drastic: Acts quickly and violently, said of cathartics

Emetic: Causes vomiting

Emmenagogue: Promotes menstruation

Emollient: Softening, soothing

Expectorant: Promotes mucus discharge from respiratory passages

Febrifuge: Reduces fever

Galactagogue: Promotes flow of milk in nursing mothers

Hemostatic: Arrests flow of blood

Hepatic: Stimulates function of liver

Hypnotic: Induces sleep

Irritant: Excites inflammation

Laxative: Produces gentle action of the bowels

Narcotic: Induces sleep or unconsciousness

Nervine: Calms nerves

Nutritive: Nourishes and sustains life

Palliative: Relieves morbid conditions without curing

Parasiticide: Destroys parasites

Parturient: Hastens labor

Pectoral: Relieves diseases of the lungs

Prophylactic: Prevents disease

Pyrogenic: Produces fever

Refrigerant: Cooling, reduces heat

Relaxant: Relieves tension, relaxes

Restorative: Brings back normal function and vitality

Rubefacient: Increases superficial circulation, producing irritation or redness

Sedative: Diminishes vital functions

Sialagogue: Stimulates secretion of saliva

Stimulant: Excites or increases vital action

Stomachic: Induces healthy action of stomach

Styptic: Stops bleeding

Sudorific: Produces perspiration

Tonic: Produces permanent increase in functional tone of the system

Toxic: Poisonous

Vermifuge: Destroys or expels worms

Vulnerary: Stimulates healing of wounds

Herbal Formula Sampler

Again I must emphasize that the following information is for suggested use only and that no claims are made for its medicinal efficacy. The herbs listed may be used singly or combined into formulas. The therapeutic value of the herb as related to the specific condition is noted. A non-specific overview of the herb's therapeutic effect can be found in the Materia Medica section. Instructions and ideas for using these sample formulas are found here, in the Common Problems/Natural Remedies section and in the Natural Therapies section. The herbs in these formulas have been traditionally and historically used in the manner described in each listing.

NOTE: Except in the case of oils which should be used in smaller quantities, ingredients are listed in alphabetical order—not in the order of proportional quantity. For more information on creating herbal formulas, see my video/workbook series, *Herbal Preparations and Natural Therapies—Creating and Using a Home Herbal Medicine Chest.*

*[P/C] indicates that some sources have listed this herb with a pregnancy caution. It should only be used after you have educated yourself about the possible side effects or if you are under the supervision of a herbalist or wholistic practitioner. For more information regarding herbs which should or should not be used in pregnancy, check the bibliography at the end of this book.

HERBAL FORMULATION TIPS

- First, look up the condition you wish to alter. You can use all the herbs listed as one complete formula, or you can custom-create your own formula by selecting only the ones you want.

- Choose the ingredients for your custom formula according to the primary effect you wish to achieve. Then add smaller quantities of the circulatory stimulants (i.e. Ginger and Cayenne) or buffers (i.e. Licorice and Marshmallow root) to round out the formula. Generally, spicy herbs are stimulating and increase circulation. These would be added to help carry the medicinal benefits of the other herbs deeper into the body. Mucilaginous herbs (those which have a viscous texture when mixed with water) are soothing. You would use these to alleviate irritation in the body, as when treating inflammation.

- When mixing your own formulas, it is helpful to add a little vegetable glycerin to prevent the ingredients from separating and to sweeten it a bit.

- 99% of the herbs listed grow in North America. I have utilized the local plants for four reasons:

  1) Plants grown in other countries are generally fumigated before being allowed entry into the US.

  2) It is easier to assure that the medicinal plants in this country have been organically grown.

  3) The plants which grow in your own bio-region are most naturally effective in healing your body.

  4) Local plants are more readily available.

- The very best medicine is made when you correctly grow, harvest and prepare the plants yourself. For most people however, this is not a possibility. Herbs can be purchased in natural food markets in the form of dried herbs, tinctures, dried plant extracts, or better yet, fresh plant extracts.

Adrenal Formula

A supportive formula for overworked, under appreciated adrenals. Use during high stress periods.

BORAGE LEAF (Borago officinalis)
Restorative for adrenal cortex, especially after cortisone or steroid treatment. Helps the body cope with intense and prolonged stress. Anti-inflammatory.

CAYENNE FRUIT (Capsicum frutescens)
Helps remedy the physiological effects of stress by equalizing circulation and strengthening the heart. Stimulant, increases assimilation and distribution of the other herbs throughout the system.

GINSENG ROOT (Panax quinquefolium)
Adaptogenic—decreases the effect of stress. Improves adrenal gland function and counteracts shrinkage of the adrenal gland due to continued stress or corticosteroid drugs. Increases capillary circulation in brain, thereby increasing mental alertness and improving quality of performance. Antidepressant. Equalizes blood pressure. Used for general exhaustion and weakness; aids digestion. Promotes longevity.

GOTU KOLA LEAF (Centella asiatica)
Used to increase mental stamina, alleviate depression and anxiety, improve memory and promote longevity. Increases energy and endurance.

LICORICE ROOT (Glycyrrhiza glabra)
Specific for adrenal gland insufficiency. Anti-inflammatory, contains constituents which are similar to cortisone. Soothing demulcent, helps to meld and balance the rest of the formula.

Allergy Formula

This formula addresses the Type I common histamine reaction which is produced by the body when it is exposed to an allergen (a substance which provokes an allergic reaction in sensitive individuals). It is useful for early onset of nasal congestion, sneezing, drippy nose and tearing eyes.

EPHEDRA (Ephedra spp.) *Mormon Tea*

Vasodilator, relieves congested sinuses; reduces spasms; stimulates circulation. Specific for asthma, bronchitis, whooping cough, hayfever. Not as intensely drying as the Chinese Ephedra.

GOLDENROD (Solidago canadensis)

Helps alleviate upper respiratory congestion by reducing inflammation, producing sweating and encouraging the elimination of excess mucus.

NETTLE (Urtica dioica)

Nutritive herb with antihistamine properties, used for childhood and nervous eczema. Rich in iron, silica, and potassium. Specific remedy for hayfever and allergies.

YERBA SANTA LEAF (Eriodictyon spp.)

Used for all forms of bronchial congestion. It stimulates the salivary and other digestive secretions, thus correcting the congestion resulting from inadequate digestion. Excellent remedy for both acute and chronic chest conditions, including asthma. Expectorant, stimulates the discharge of mucus. Opens air passages; mild decongestant.

Aloe Burn Spray Formula

Used for sunburn, windburn and common household burns.
Can also be used as an antiseptic spray.

ALOE (Aloe vera) [P/C, internally]

Applied fresh or as a prepared juice to alleviate the pain and inflammation of burns and wounds; astringent. Known as "Nature's bandaid." Speeds healing.

CALENDULA FLOWER (Calendula officinalis)

Anti-inflammatory; astringent; styptic; used topically for wounds, ulcers, burns, abscesses.

COMFREY ROOT/LEAF (Symphytum officinalis) [external]

Demulcent, soothes irritation, promotes healing.

LAVENDER OIL

Antiseptic, soothing, healing.

Anti-Fungal Formula

For internal or external fungal infections such as Candidiasis.

ANGELICA ROOT (Angelica spp.)
Anti-fungal.

BLACK WALNUT HULLS (Juglans nigra)
Antifungal, (for Candida, athlete's foot, ringworm, etc.); astringent, used for skin eruptions.

CALENDULA FLOWER (Calendula officinalis)
Anti-inflammatory; astringent; antifungal.

COLTSFOOT (Tussilago farfara)
Astringent, anti-inflammatory. Externally for sores, ulcers and fungal infections.

DESERT WILLOW LEAF/BARK (Chilopsis linearis)
Anti-fungal. Used to treat Candida albicans, specifically the symptoms of candida supra-infections which are abundant after antibiotic therapy, i.e. indigestion, loose stools, hemorrhoids, rectal aching, foul burping, etc.

GARLIC BULB/SEED (Allium sativum)
Anti-fungal; antibiotic; anti-microbial; antiseptic.

GOLDENROD (Solidago virgauria)
Anti-inflammatory; anti-fungal.

PAU D' ARCO (Tabebuia impetiginosa)
Blood cleanser; anti-fungal; used for Candida.

ROSEMARY LEAF (Rosmarinus officinalis)
Anti-bacterial; anti-fungal.

SPILANTHES (Spilanthes oleracea)
Anti-fungal, anti-bacterial; used specifically for Candidiasis.

USNEA LICHEN (Usnea spp.)
Strong antibiotic; anti-fungal; for internal infections, infected wounds.

Anti-Fungal External Spray Formula

*For external fungal infections such as Athlete's foot,
Ringworm and Jock itch.*

BLACK WALNUT HULLS (Juglans nigra)
Antifungal, astringent, used for skin eruptions.

CALENDULA FLOWER (Calendula officinalis)
Anti-inflammatory; astringent; styptic; antifungal.

GARLIC BULB/SEED (Allium sativum)
Anti-fungal; antibiotic; anti-microbial; antiseptic; antiviral; anthelmintic.

PAU D' ARCO (Tabebuia impetiginosa)
Blood cleanser; anti-fungal; used for candida.

SPILANTHES (Spilanthes oleracea)
Anti-fungal; anti-bacterial; used for Candidiasis. Relieves pain.

USNEA LICHEN (Usnea spp.)
Strong antibiotic; anti-viral; anti-fungal.

CLARY SAGE ESSENTIAL OIL (Salvia sclarea)
Anti-fungal.

TEA TREE OIL (Melaleuca alternifolia)
Anti-fungal; antiseptic; vulnerary; speeds healing.

Antiseptic Spray Formula

For prevention of infection in minor cuts and scrapes or as a spray for sprains and strains.

CALENDULA FLOWER (Calendula officinalis)
Anti-inflammatory; astringent; styptic; antifungal; topically for wounds, ulcers, burns, abscesses.

CAYENNE FRUIT (Capsicum frutescens)
Antiseptic. Styptic. (Yes, it stings).

CHAPARRAL LEAF (Larrea tridentata)
Antibiotic; anti-viral; antiseptic; specific for infections.

ECHINACEA ROOT (Echinacea angustifolia)
Antiseptic; anti-microbial; anti-viral; stimulates immune response.

GOLDENSEAL ROOT (Hydrastis canadensis)
Antiseptic, used topically for infection, sore throat, ulceration.

MYRRH GUM (Commiphora myrrha)
Used externally on cuts and abrasions, forms natural bandaid. Antiseptic; anti-microbial; astringent. Used for mouth ulcers, sore throat, gingivitis, pyorrhea.

EUCALYPTUS OIL (Eucalyptus citriodora)
Antiseptic, bactericide, disinfectant.

Antiviral Formula

For herpes, shingles, flu, warts and other viruses. Can be taken internally or applied externally.

BONESET (Eupatorium perfoliatum)
For flu symptoms, aches and pains; clears mucus congestion; reduces fevers and muscular rheumatism.

CHAPARRAL LEAF (Larrea tridentata)
Blood cleanser; antibiotic; anti-viral; antiseptic; specific for infections, sluggish liver, skin problems.

ECHINACEA ROOT (Echinacea angustifolia)
Immune stimulant; antiseptic; anti-microbial; anti-viral; used for sore throats, flu, colds, infections, allergies.

GINGER ROOT (Asarum canadense)
Helps break fevers by causing the body to sweat; stimulant; aids in utilization of other herbs.

LOMATIUM ROOT (Lomatium dissectum)
Antiviral; immune stimulant; for colds, flu, viral sore throats, respiratory infections and congestion.

OSHA' ROOT (Ligusticum porterii)
Strong antiviral, used for herpes, sore throat, colds, flu; bronchial expectorant; immune stimulating properties.

ST. JOHN'S WORT (Hypericum perforatum)
Immune system stimulant; for retro-viral infections; expectorant; anti-bacterial.

TRONADORA (Tecoma stans)
Anti-viral, particularly helpful for herpes simplex.

USNEA LICHEN (Usnea spp.)
Strong antibiotic; antiviral; for internal infections, strep, staph, trichomonas, etc., infected wounds. Also used for pneumonia, TB and Lupus.

Asthma Formula

Relaxing, decongestant formula.

BUTTERBUR (Petasites hybridus)
Muscle relaxant, mild febrifuge.

COLTSFOOT (Tussilago farfara)
Soothing expectorant, demulcent, antispasmodic, astringent, anti-inflammatory. For irritating coughs, bronchitis, asthma, laryngitis, throat catarrh.

ELECAMPANE ROOT (Inula helenium)
Expectorant; diaphoretic; anti-bacterial; anti-tussive; stomachic; for irritating bronchial coughs, bronchitis, emphysema, asthma and bronchitic asthma.

EPHEDRA (Ephedra spp.) *Mormon Tea*
Vasodilator; antispasmodic; hypertensive; circulatory stimulant; used for asthma, bronchitis, whooping cough, hayfever; opens air passages.

INMORTAL ROOT (Asclepius asperula)
Bronchial dilator; stimulates lymph drainage from the lungs. Used for asthma, pleurisy, bronchitis, lung infections. Laxative, diaphoretic, mild cardiac tonic.

LOBELIA HERB (Lobelia inflata)
Respiratory stimulant; anti-asthmatic; anti-emetic (small dose), emetic (large dose). Used for bronchitis and bronchitic asthma, whooping cough, muscular cramping and pain.

PEPPERMINT LEAF (Mentha piperita)
For upset stomach, heartburn, nausea, colds, flu, congestion, nervous headache and agitation. Adds flavor to other herbs.

WILD CHERRY BARK (Prunus serotina)
Expectorant, anti-tussive, astringent, sedative, digestive bitter. Used for irritating coughs, bronchitis and asthma.

YERBA SANTA LEAF (Eriodycton spp.)
Expectorant; bronchial dilator; mild decongestant, for chest colds, asthma, hayfever, bronchitis.

Bronchial Formula

For bronchitis, deep chest inflammation and congestion.

COLTSFOOT (Tussilago farfara)
Soothing expectorant, demulcent, antispasmodic, astringent, anti-inflammatory. Helps alleviate irritating coughs, bronchitis, laryngitis, throat catarrh.

ELECAMPANE ROOT (Inula helenium)
Expectorant; diaphoretic; anti-bacterial; anti-tussive; for irritating bronchial coughs, bronchitis, and bronchitic asthma.

LICORICE ROOT (Glycyrrhiza glabra)
Demulcent; expectorant for coughs and respiratory congestion; anti-inflammatory; laxative.

PEPPERMINT LEAF (Mentha piperita)
Decongestant. Mild diaphoretic. Digestive herb.

PLEURISY ROOT (Asclepias tuberosa)
Reduces inflammation and encourages expectoration.

STILLINGIA ROOT (Stillingia sylvatica)
Stimulating expectorant. Small dose laxative and diuretic; large dose cathartic and emetic.

WILD CHERRY BARK (Prunus serotina)
Expectorant, anti-tussive, astringent, sedative, digestive bitter. Used for irritating coughs, bronchitis and asthma.

YERBA SANTA LEAF (Eriodictyon spp.)
Expectorant; bronchial dilator; mild decongestant, for chest colds, asthma, hayfever, bronchitis.

Bug Spray Formula

To discourage insects from trespassing on your body. The following essential oils are all known for their insect repellant properties.

CITRONELLA (Ceylonese or Javanese)

EUCALYPTUS (Eucalyptus citriodora)

LAVENDER (Lavandula officinalis)

PENNYROYAL (Mentha pelugium)

Children's Calming Glycerite Formula

Glycerites are made by extracting the herbs in vegetable glycerin and distilled water. They do not contain the full range of medicinal constituents, but still have mild therapeutic effects. Makes bitter tasting extracts more palatable for children when used as a base. This formula is particularly useful to soothe children on airplanes and in other stressful situations. It is also very helpful to alleviate crankiness during the teething period.

ALFALFA (Medicago sativa)
Nutritive herb with high mineral and vitamin content, including vitamin K and iron.

CATNIP HERB (Nepeta cataria)
For indigestion, flatulence and colic; mild astringent, specific for childhood fevers and diarrhea.

CHAMOMILE FLOWER (Matricaria recutita)
Reduces fever and calms restlessness. Mild pain reliever, helps relieve colic, dispel gas.

FENNEL SEED (Foeniculum vulgare)
Aids digestion; relieves flatulence and colic; expels mucous; flavoring agent; increases digestibility of other herbs.

LEMON BALM (Melissa officinalis)
Very useful in reducing fevers during colds and flu since it induces mild perspiration. Aids digestion, reduces flatulence.

LICORICE ROOT (Glycyrrhiza glabra)
Soothing demulcent; mild laxative.

RED RASPBERRY LEAF (Rhubus idaeus)
Nutritive, relieves nausea. Remedy for childhood diarrhea.

ROSEHIPS (Rosa canina)
Nutritive, mild diuretic and laxative, mild astringent. Good source of vitamin C. Used for colds, flu, general debility and exhaustion, constipation.

Clear Eyes Formula

*An **internal** formula for eye strain and infections.*
Do not place in eyes.

BILBERRY (Vaccinum myrtillus)
Astringent, antiseptic, absorptive. Used to enhance vision when taken for long periods of time.

ECHINACEA ROOT (Echinacea angustifolia)
Powerful immune stimulant; antiseptic; anti-microbial; anti-viral. Helps the body combat infections.

EYEBRIGHT HERB (Euphrasia officinalis)
Anti-catarrhal, astringent, anti-inflammatory. Internally for sinusitis, nasal congestion, eye inflammations.

GOLDENSEAL ROOT (Hydrastis canadensis)
Antiseptic, used for infections. Should not be taken daily for more than a week or so as overuse can stress the liver.

RED RASPBERRY LEAF (Rhubus idaeus)
Nutritive; astringent; helps strengthen eyes.

RED ROOT (Ceanothus americana)
Stimulates lymphatic function, helping to carry toxins out of the body.

USNEA LICHEN (Usnea spp.)
Strong antibiotic; antiviral; antifungal; for internal infections, staph, etc., infected wounds.

Clear Thought Formula

To increase mental clarity; also helpful when adjusting to higher altitudes.

CAYENNE FRUIT (Capsicum frutescens)
Equalizes circulation; for cold hands and feet; strengthens heart; stimulant.

GINKGO LEAF (Ginkgo biloba)
Stimulates cerebral circulation and oxygenation, mental clarity and alertness, improves memory.

GINSENG ROOT (Panax quinquefolium)
Adaptogenic, decreases the effect of stress. Increases capillary circulation in brain; reproductive tonic; anti-depressant; equalizes blood pressure. Used for general exhaustion and weakness; aids digestion. Promotes longevity.

GOTU KOLA LEAF (Centella asiatica)
Used to increase mental stamina, alleviate depression and anxiety, improve memory and promote longevity. Increases energy and endurance.

LICORICE ROOT (Glycyrrhiza glabra)
Supports adrenal glands.

Computer Stress Formula

To alleviate the effects of computer radiation exposure, metabolic depression, eyestrain, nervous tension, lack of libido and mental fatigue.

BLADDERWRACK (Fucus vesiculosus)
Thyroid balancer, specific in treating obesity associated with underactive thyroid.

DANDELION ROOT/LEAF (Taraxacum officinale)
Blood cleanser; powerful and safe diuretic, high in potassium. Mild laxative, aids weight loss, lowers cholesterol and blood pressure.

ECHINACEA ROOT (Echinacea angustifolia)
Powerful immune stimulant; antiseptic; anti-microbial; anti-viral.

EYEBRIGHT HERB (Euphrasia officinalis)
Helps strengthen eyes, decreases eyestrain.

GINKGO LEAF (Ginkgo biloba)
Stimulates cerebral circulation and oxygenation, mental clarity and alertness, improves memory.

GOTU KOLA LEAF (Centella asiatica)
Used to increase mental stamina, alleviate depression and anxiety, improve memory and promote longevity. Increases energy and endurance.

KELP (Nereocystis luetkeana)
Radiation protective properties. Reduces amount of strontium-90 absorbed by bone tissue by 50-85%.

LICORICE ROOT (Glycyrrhiza glabra)
Supports adrenal gland; anti-inflammatory; laxative.

OAT SEED (Avena sativa)
Antispasmodic; soothes and supports nervous system; for depression, hysteria, irritation and anxiety.

Cough Calm Formula

*An antispasmodic, mildly expectorant formula for the dry, annoying,
unproductive cough that prevents restful sleep.*

BLUE VERVAIN (Verbena spp.)
Soothes cranky children; sedative; diaphoretic; febrifuge; antispasmodic;
mild analgesic.

CAYENNE FRUIT (Capsicum frutescens)
Stimulant; antiseptic, used as gargle for persistent cough.

COLTSFOOT (Tussilago farfara)
Soothing expectorant; demulcent; antispasmodic; astringent; anti-inflammatory. For irritating coughs, bronchitis, asthma, laryngitis, throat
catarrh.

ELECAMPANE ROOT (Inula helenium)
Expectorant; diaphoretic; antibacterial; anti-tussive; stomachic. Used
for irritating bronchial coughs, bronchitis, emphysema, asthma and
bronchitic asthma.

JAMAICAN DOGWOOD (Piscidia erythrina)
Sedative; anodyne; smooth muscle antispasmodic. For insomnia, neuralgia. Relieves coughing, reduces fevers.

LICORICE ROOT (Glycyrrhiza glabra)
Demulcent; expectorant for coughs and respiratory congestion; anti-
inflammatory; laxative.

LOBELIA HERB (Lobelia inflata)
Respiratory stimulant; anti-spasmodic.

Cramp Relief Formula

To relieve menstrual and muscular cramping.

BLACK COHOSH ROOT (Cimicifuga racemosa) [P/C]
Antispasmodic, used for menstrual cramping, coughs, muscle spasms; emmenagogue; relieves hot flashes in menopausal women; mild sedative.

CRAMP BARK (Viburnum opulus)
Relaxes muscle tension and spasms, ovarian and uterine cramps. Used to prevent threatened miscarriage.

LOBELIA HERB (Lobelia inflata)
Anti-emetic (small dose), emetic (large dose); Used for muscular cramping and pain.

VALERIAN ROOT (Valeriana officinalis)
Powerful nervine, used for tension, anxiety, insomnia, emotional stress, intestinal colic, menstrual cramps, migraine headache and rheumatic pain.

Detox Formula

A cleansing formula which gently encourages the elimination of excess waste.

ANISE SEED (Pimpinella anisum)
Eases indigestion, flatulence and colic. Antispasmodic and expectorant.

BUCKTHORN BARK (Rhamnus frangula)
Moderately strong laxative, very useful in chronic constipation. Must be dried before use to avoid intestinal cramping and nausea.

BURDOCK ROOT (Arctium lappa)
Blood cleanser, used for skin eruptions, dry/scaly skin conditions; digestive stimulant.

DANDELION ROOT/LEAF (Taraxacum officinale)
Blood cleanser; powerful and safe diuretic; high in potassium; cholagogue, for inflammation and congestion of the liver and gall bladder, congestive jaundice. Mild laxative, aids weight loss, lowers cholesterol and blood pressure.

ECHINACEA ROOT (Echinacea angustifolia)
Powerful immune stimulant; antiseptic; anti-microbial; anti-viral; used for sore throats, flu, colds, infections, allergies.

OREGON GRAPE ROOT (Mahonia repens)
Liver and blood cleanser; cholagogue; anti-bacterial. Stimulates digestion and absorption. Used for sluggish liver, hangovers, acne, eczema.

STILLINGIA ROOT (Stillingia sylvatica)
Blood cleanser, used for skin disorders. Small dose laxative and diuretic, large dose cathartic and emetic.

STONE ROOT (Collinsonia canadensis)
Strong diuretic, helps prevent and dissolve urinary stones and gravel.

WAHOO (Euonymus atropurpureus)
Primary liver decongestant, bile stimulant; used for jaundice, gallbladder pain and inflammation, constipation.

YARROW FLOWERS (Achillea millefolium)
Diaphoretic, helps release toxic waste and reduce fevers.

Digestive Formula

*Carminative and bitter herbs to stimulate digestion and reduce flatulence.
Best taken with meals.*

ALFALFA (Medicago sativa)
Nutritive herb with high mineral and vitamin content including Vit. K
and iron.

ANISE SEED (Pimpinella anisum)
Aids digestion, reduces flatulence and colic. Antispasmodic.

CAYENNE FRUIT (Capsicum frutescens)
Equalizes circulation; stimulant; carminative.

DILL SEED (Anethum graveolens)
Carminative, used to prevent flatulence and colic, especially in children.

FENNEL SEED (Foeniculum vulgare)
Aids digestion; relieves flatulence and colic; expels mucous; aids weight
loss; flavoring agent; increases digestibility of other herbs.

GENTIAN ROOT (Gentiana lutea)
Bitter, promotes production of gastric juices and bile. For sluggish
digestion, dyspepsia and flatulence. Restores appetite lost during morning sickness.

GINGER ROOT (Asarum canadense)
Carminative; aids in utilization of other herbs. Stimulant.

MEADOWSWEET (Filipendula ulmaria)
Digestive herb, antacid. Used for heartburn, nausea, gastritis, hyper-
acidity, peptic ulcers. Mild astringent, used for diarrhea in children.
Anti-inflammatory.

PEPPERMINT LEAF (Mentha piperita)
For upset stomach, heartburn, nausea, colds, flu, congestion, nervous
headache and agitation, also diarrhea and flatulence. Adds flavor to
other herbs.

Diuretic Formula

To decrease water retention by increasing the flow of urine.

BURDOCK SEED (Arctium lappa)
Diuretic, kidney tonic, demulcent.

CHICKWEED HERB (Stellaria media)
Nutritive; restorative; demulcent; diuretic.

CORN SILK (Zea mays)
Soothing diuretic, for renal & urinary irritation; used for bedwetting, cystitis, urethritis, prostatitis.

CRANBERRY (Vaccinium oxycoccus)
Diuretic and urinary antiseptic; for kidney and bladder infections.

DANDELION ROOT/LEAF (Taraxacum officinale)
Powerful and safe diuretic, high in potassium. Mild laxative, aids weight loss.

GOLDENROD (Solidago virgauria)
Anti-inflammatory; urinary antiseptic; diuretic; diaphoretic; astringent.

PARSLEY LEAF/ROOT (Petroselenum crispum) [P/C]
Diuretic, antispasmodic.

STONE ROOT (Collinsonia canadensis)
Strong diuretic, helps prevent and dissolve urinary stones and gravel.

UVA URSI (Arcostaphylos uva-ursi)
Urinary antiseptic; anti-microbial; for cystitis, urethritis, prostatitis, nephritis. Antilithic, used for kidney and bladder stones.

Eczema Formula

For dry, scaly, itchy skin.

ALFALFA (Medicago sativa)
Nutritive herb with high mineral and vitamin content including Vit. K and iron; mild diuretic.

BURDOCK ROOT (Arctium lappa)
Blood cleanser, used for skin eruptions, dry/scaly skin conditions; digestive stimulant.

CHAPARRAL LEAF (Larrea tridentata)
Blood cleanser, antioxidant; antibiotic; anti-viral; antiseptic; specific for infections, sluggish liver, skin problems.

FIGWORT HERB (Scrophularia spp.)
Used internally and topically for eczema, scrofula, cradle cap, psoriasis, itching and irritated skin. *Avoid in cases of tachycardia.*

HORSETAIL HERB (Equisetum arvense)
High in silica and calcium, used to strengthen hair, skin and nails.

NETTLE (Urtica dioica)
Nutritive herb, specific for childhood and nervous eczema. Rich in iron, silica, and potassium. Diuretic.

Expectorant Formula

To help move excess mucus out of the body, while soothing irritated membranes.

BLOODROOT (Sanguinaria canadensis)
Expectorant. For chronic bronchitis, croup, laryngitis.

BONESET (Eupatorium perfoliatum)
For flu symptoms, aches and pains; clears mucus congestion; reduces fevers.

COLTSFOOT (Tussilago farfara)
Soothing expectorant, demulcent, antispasmodic, astringent, anti-inflammatory. For irritating coughs, bronchitis, asthma laryngitis, throat catarrh.

GINGER ROOT (Asarum canadense)
Used for nausea. Diaphoretic, helps break fevers; stimulant; aids in utilization of other herbs.

GRINDELIA BUDS/FLOWERS (Grindelia spp.)
Expectorant; anti-spasmodic; for bronchitis, sinus congestion.

INMORTAL ROOT (Asclepius asperula)
Bronchial dilator; stimulates lymph drainage from the lungs. Used for asthma, pleurisy, bronchitis, lung infections. Laxative, diaphoretic.

LICORICE ROOT (Glycyrrhiza glabra)
Demulcent; expectorant. For coughs and respiratory congestion; anti-inflammatory; laxative.

MULLEIN LEAF (Verbascum thapsus)
Expectorant; demulcent; reduces respiratory inflammation.

OSHA' ROOT (Ligusticum porterii)
Strong antiviral, used for herpes, sore throat, colds, flu; bronchial expectorant; immune stimulating properties.

PLEURISY ROOT (Asclepias tuberosa)
Respiratory infections, bronchitis, pleurisy, pneumonia, flu. Reduces inflammation and encourages expectoration.

Female Glandular Formula

Formulated to gently balance female glandular function.
Warning—has been known to increase libido.

BLACK COHOSH ROOT (Cimicifuga racemosa) [P/C]
Antispasmodic, used for menstrual cramping; emmenagogue; relieves hot flashes in menopausal women; mild sedative.

CHASTE BERRY (Vitex agnus castus)
Reproductive tonic, stimulates and normalizes pituitary function. For menstrual cramps, PMS, menopause, post birth control pill rebalancing.

DANDELION ROOT/LEAF (Taraxacum officinale)
Blood cleanser; powerful and safe diuretic, high in potassium. Mild laxative, aids weight loss, lowers cholesterol and blood pressure.

DONG QUAI ROOT (Angelica sinensis)
Female hormone regulator, alleviates cramping and pre-menstrual distress.

HOPS STROBILE (Humulus lupus)
Sedative; hypnotic. Used for anxiety, tension, insomnia. Reduces nervous irritability, promotes restful sleep.

RHUBARB (Rheum palmatum)
Stomachic, astringent, small doses to relieve diarrhea, larger doses laxative.

SQUAWVINE/PARTRIDGE BERRY (Mitchella repens)
Uterine tonic; promotes easy labor, eases menstrual cramping, mild nervine, improves digestion.

Fresh Breath Gum Tonic

Drop this antiseptic, astringent formula on your toothbrush and brush up under your gums to cleanse and strengthen the tissue. Freshens breath.

BLOODROOT (Sanguinaria canadensis)
Alleviates mouth sores and reduces dental plaque.

CALENDULA FLOWER (Calendula officinalis)
Anti-inflammatory; astringent; styptic; antifungal. Use topically for wounds, ulcerations, abscesses.

MYRRH GUM (Commiphora myrrha)
Antiseptic; anti-microbial; astringent. Used for mouth ulcers, sore throat, gingivitis, pyorrhea.

PEPPERMINT LEAF (Mentha piperita)
Cooling, astringent. Adds flavor to other herbs.

POTENTILLA (Potentilla spp.)
Astringent mouthwash and gargle for sore throats or gum inflammation.

WHITE OAK BARK (Quercus alba)
Astringent, used for bleeding or ulcerated gums. Strengthens capillaries. Helps tighten teeth.

WILD YAM ROOT (Dioscorea spp.)
Anti-inflammatory.

PEPPERMINT AND CINNAMON OILS
For flavor, and to freshen breath.

Healthy Skin Formula

A cleansing and supportive formula for internal or external use in acne, eczema, and easily irritated skin.

ALFALFA (Medicago sativa)
Nutritive herb with high mineral and vitamin content including Vit. K and iron; mild diuretic.

BLUE FLAG ROOT (Iris versicolor)
Liver purgative; blood purifier; cathartic; sialagogue; diuretic. For constipation and biliousness, eruptive skin conditions.

BURDOCK ROOT (Arctium lappa)
Blood cleanser, used for skin eruptions, dry/scaly skin conditions; digestive stimulant.

HORSETAIL HERB (Equisetum arvense)
High in silica and calcium, used to strengthen hair, skin and nails.

NETTLE (Urtica dioica)
Nutritive herb, specific for childhood and nervous eczema. Rich in iron, silica, and potassium. For anemia. Diuretic; antihistamine.

OAT SEED (Avena sativa)
Antispasmodic; soothes and supports nervous system. Calms irritation and anxiety.

OREGON GRAPE ROOT (Mahonia repens)
Liver and blood cleanser; cholagogue; anti-bacterial. Stimulates digestion and absorption. Used for sluggish liver, acne, eczema.

RED CLOVER FLOWERS (Trifolium pratense)
Blood cleanser; nutritive; used for childhood eczema, psoriasis, ulcers, inflammation and infection. Principal ingredient of the Hoxey cancer formula.

Immune Strengthening Formula

An immune stimulant formula to help prevent susceptibility to disease. Best taken when you know you've been exposed to the latest grunge that's been going around, before it has developed into full-blown symptoms. Echinacea seems to work best when it is not over-utilized.

ECHINACEA ROOT (Echinacea angustifolia)
Powerful immune stimulant; antiseptic; anti-microbial; anti-viral; used for sore throats, flu, colds, infections, allergies.

GINSENG ROOT (Panax quinquefolium)
Adaptogenic, decreases the effect of stress. Increases capillary circulation in brain; reproductive tonic; anti-depressant; equalizes blood pressure. Used for general exhaustion and weakness; aids digestion. Promotes longevity.

LOMATIUM ROOT (Lomatium dissectum)
Antiviral; immune stimulant; for colds, flu, viral sore throats, respiratory infections and congestion.

OSHA' ROOT (Ligusticum porterii)
Strong antiviral, used for herpes, sore throat, colds, flu; bronchial expectorant with immune stimulating properties.

ST. JOHN'S WORT (Hypericum perforatum)
Extract used internally as an immune system stimulant; for retro-viral infections; expectorant; anti-bacterial, speeds wound and burn healing; anti-depressant.

Infection Formula

(This is the formula to use when you know you've definitely "got the bug" that's been flying around. The sooner you take care of it, the easier it will be to get rid of. The first sniffle is the most appropriate time to nip it in the bud.)

BONESET (Eupatorium perfoliatum)
For flu symptoms, aches and pains; clears mucus congestion; reduces fevers; muscular rheumatism.

CAYENNE FRUIT (Capsicum frutescens)
Equalizes circulation; stimulant; styptic. Antiseptic, used as a gargle for persistent cough and laryngitis.

CHAMOMILE FLOWER (Matricaria recutita)
Sedative, antispasmodic, anodyne. Children's herb, especially for fever and restlessness. Mouthwash for gingivitis.

ECHINACEA ROOT (Echinacea angustifolia)
Powerful immune stimulant; antiseptic; anti-microbial; anti-viral; used for sore throats, flu, colds, infections, allergies.

OREGON GRAPE ROOT (Mahonia repens)
Liver and blood cleanser; cholagogue; anti-bacterial. Stimulates digestion and absorption.

OSHA' ROOT (Ligusticum porterii)
Strong antiviral, used for herpes, sore throat, colds, flu; bronchial expectorant with immune stimulating properties.

RED ROOT (Ceanothus americana)
Stimulates lymphatic system. Used for tonsillitis, sore throat, enlarged lymph nodes and spleen, fibrous cysts.

USNEA LICHEN (Usnea spp.)
Strong antibiotic; antiviral; antifungal; for internal infections, strep, staph, trichomonas, etc., infected wounds. Also used for pneumonia, TB and Lupus.

Intestinal Fiber Maintenance Formula

Healthy intestines are vital to health in the rest of the body. Proper digestion, assimilation and elimination are essential for balanced metabolism and a strong immune system. This formula is best made with freshly ground seeds and should be refrigerated so the oils in the seeds do not go rancid. Keep it tightly closed when not in use. All the ingredients must be organically grown and cold processed. To use this formula, it is best to keep a small covered container handy to mix it in. Add one rounded teaspoon to 8 ounces of water or juice, shake well and drink immediately, because it thickens quickly. Follow with another glass of water and drink water throughout the day. This formula should be an integral part of any detoxification or weight loss program as well as daily maintenance. Different dietary fibers produce specific metabolic effects in the body. This formula provides a full spectrum of these fibers with herbal catalysts for maximum benefit.

ALFALFA LEAF (Medicago sativa)
Anti-bacterial. High fiber, binds and neutralizes substances that are carcinogenic to the colon.

APPLE PECTIN
Soft bulking agent which binds with bile acids. Used to reduce blood pressure and cholesterol.

BENTONITE CLAY
Highly absorbent. Helps "draw" impacted matter from the sides of the intestinal wall, further enhancing the detoxifying effect of the rest of the formula.

BUCKTHORN BARK (Rhamnus frangula)
Moderately strong laxative, very useful in chronic constipation.

BUTTERNUT BARK (Juglans cinerea)
Mild laxative; hepatic decongestant; vermifuge. Used to treat dysentery.

CASCARA SAGRADA BARK (Rhamnus purshiana) [P/C]
Laxative, mild liver stimulant, bitter tonic.

CAYENNE FRUIT (Capsicum frutescens)
Equalizes circulation; stimulant; carminative; styptic, antiseptic.

DANDELION ROOT/LEAF (Taraxacum officinale)
Mild laxative, liver/gall bladder decongestant, aids weight loss, lowers cholesterol and blood pressure. High in potassium.

FLAX SEED (Linum usitatissimum)
Excellent bulking agent which cleanses and lubricates digestive tract.

GARLIC BULB/SEED (Allium sativum)
Antibiotic; anti-microbial; antiseptic; antiviral; anthelmintic. Helps reduce blood pressure and cholesterol.

GOTU KOLA (Centella asiatica)
Tonic, blood purifier, antispasmodic. Increases circulation, decreases fatigue. Helps heal ulcerated tissue.

JERUSALEM ARTICHOKE (Helianthus annuus)
Helps stimulate the growth of healthy intestinal flora.

KELP (Nereocystis luetkeana)
Used for radiation detoxification and to balance metabolism. Reduces amount of strontium-90 absorbed by bone tissue by 50-85%.

LACTOBACILLIS ACIDOPHILUS AND B. BIFIDUM/ LONGUM
Restores the balance of healthy intestinal flora, thus inhibiting the growth of putrefactive bacteria.

OAT BRAN FIBER (Avena sativa)
Bulking agent, helps reduce cholesterol. Calming.

PSYLLIUM SEED (Plantago ovata)
Commonly called the intestinal janitor, softly "scrubs" the sides of the intestinal wall for maximum cleansing effect.

Remember to keep this formula refrigerated for maximum benefit!

Iron Rich Formula

Increases the body's ability to utilize oxygen, thus increasing energy. Iron is essential for growth in children and resistance to disease. Iron is reduced in the body during infections, stress and the menstrual flow, and by the dietary consumption of carbonated soft drinks, alcohol, aspirin, coffee and black tea. Iron deficiency is common in people who have either chronic herpes infections or candidiasis. It is recognized as one of the most prevalent mineral deficiencies in humans. Iron deficiency is indicated in chronic fatigue, lethargy, listlessness, depression, sleeplessness, brittle hair and fingernails. It also decreases the ability to tolerate cold weather.

BURDOCK ROOT (Arctium lappa)
Helps detoxify the bloodstream. Abundance of iron and insulin makes it of special value to the blood. Clears the kidneys of excess wastes and uric acid by increasing the flow of urine. Used for skin eruptions, dry/scaly skin conditions; increases digestion.

CHICKWEED HERB (Stellaria media)
A medicinal food which is high in B-Complex vitamins, ascorbic acid, iron, calcium, sodium, zinc, lecithin and molybdenum. Used to build the blood and restore nutritional balance. Chickweed also assists in regulating the thyroid and has been used in weight loss programs. Increases cell membrane permeability, thus increasing the absorption of nutrients.

MULLEIN LEAF (Verbascum thapsus)
One of the highest herbal sources of bio-available iron. Demulcent, soothing to the gastro-intestinal tract.

NETTLE (Urtica dioica)
Nutritive herb, specific for childhood and nervous eczema. Rich in iron, silica, and potassium. Used to correct anemia.

YELLOW DOCK ROOT (Rumex crispus)
Nutritive tonic, aids in the assimilation of iron. Mild laxative, stimulates the flow of bile and aids fat digestion.

Itch-Ease Spray Formula

Relieves itching of insect bites, poison ivy, poison oak, etc.

ECHINACEA ROOT (Echinacea angustifolia)
Antiseptic; anti-microbial.

GRINDELIA BUDS/FLOWERS (Grindelia spp.)
Relieves swelling, itching, and pain of poison oak/ivy and insect bites.

JEWELWEED (Impatiens aurens)
EXTERNAL USE. Used topically to reduce the itching and inflammation of skin irritating plants such as poison ivy.

NETTLE (Urtica dioica)
Nutritive herb, specific for childhood and nervous eczema. Rich in iron, silica, and potassium. Antihistamine, reduces inflammation and itching.

PLANTAIN LEAF (Plantago spp.)
Astringent; used for external wounds and sores, insect bites.

POTENTILLA (Potentilla spp.)
Astringent, used for abrasions, sunburn, poison oak.

Joint Formula

For the stiffness and soreness associated with arthritis. Increases lymphatic drainage.

ECHINACEA ROOT (Echinacea angustifolia)
Powerful immune stimulant; aids lymphatic drainage; used for sore throats, flu, colds, infections, allergies.

MEADOWSWEET (Filipendula ulmaria)
Digestive herb, antacid. Used for heartburn, nausea, gastritis, hyper-acidity, peptic ulcers. Mild astringent. Diaphoretic, anti-inflammatory, reduces fever and pain.

RED ROOT (Ceanothus americana)
Stimulates lymphatic and interstitial fluid circulation. Aids in the transport of nutrients and the elimination of waste products.

WILD YAM ROOT (Dioscorea spp.)
Antispasmodic; anti-inflammatory; helps alleviate the pain and swelling of rheumatoid arthritis.

YERBA MANSA ROOT (Anemopsis californica)
Soothing to mucus membranes, used for catarrh, aids digestion.

Kidney/Bladder Formula

Antiseptic and demulcent herbs to help alleviate urinary irritation and promote healing. Mild diuretic.

BURDOCK ROOT (Arctium lappa)
Blood cleanser, digestive stimulant.

CORN SILK (Zea mays)
Soothing diuretic, for renal & urinary irritation; used for bedwetting, cystitis, urethritis, prostatitis.

COUCHGRASS ROOT (Agropyron repens)
Demulcent; anti-microbial; antilithic; for cystitis, urethritis, prostatitis, kidney stones and gravel.

CRANBERRY (Vaccinium oxycoccus)
Diuretic and urinary antiseptic; for kidney and bladder infections.

GOLDENROD (Solidago virgauria)
Anti-inflammatory; urinary antiseptic; diuretic; diaphoretic; expectorant, astringent. For cystitis, urethritis, upper respiratory catarrh, diarrhea and internal hemorrhage.

GRAVEL ROOT (Eupatorium purpureum)
For kidney and urinary infections and stones; prostatitis; pelvic inflammatory disease; painful menses; rheumatism and gout.

MARSHMALLOW ROOT (Althaea officinalis)
Demulcent, soothes inflamed membranes.

PIPSISSEWA (Chimaphila umbellata)
Diuretic, used for chronic kidney weakness, nephritis, bladder stones and rheumatism.

UVA URSI (Arcostaphylos uva-ursi)
Urinary antiseptic; anti-microbial; for cystitis, urethritis, prostatitis, nephritis. Antilithic, used for kidney and bladder stones.

Laxative Formula

A balance of cleansing and soothing herbs to tone the lower intestine and promote effective elimination.

ANISE SEED (Pimpinella anisum)
Eases indigestion, flatulence and colic. Antispasmodic.

BARBERRY ROOT (Berberis fendleri) [P/C]
Digestive and appetite stimulant; stimulates bile flow and liver function; refrigerant, reduces fevers; antiseptic.

BUCKTHORN BARK (Rhamnus frangula)
Moderately strong laxative, very useful in chronic constipation. Must be dried before use to avoid intestinal cramping and nausea.

DANDELION ROOT/LEAF (Taraxacum officinale)
Blood cleanser; powerful and safe diuretic, high in potassium; stimulates flow of bile, for inflammation and congestion of the liver and gall bladder. Mild laxative, aids weight loss, lowers cholesterol and blood pressure.

ECHINACEA ROOT (Echinacea angustifolia)
Immune stimulant; antiseptic; anti-microbial; anti-viral.

LICORICE ROOT (Glycyrrhiza glabra)
Demulcent; anti-inflammatory; laxative.

MARSHMALLOW ROOT (Althaea officinalis)
Soothing demulcent, reduces gastro-intestinal inflammation.

POTENTILLA (Potentilla spp.)
Astringent. Used for gastro-intestinal ulcers.

RHUBARB ROOT (Rheum palmatum) [P/C]
Stomachic, astringent, small doses to relieve diarrhea, larger doses laxative.

WILD YAM ROOT (Dioscorea spp.)
Antispasmodic; carminative; anti-inflammatory; hepatic; cholagogue; diaphoretic. Used for intestinal colic, diverticulitis, flatulence.

Liver Formula

Cleansing and stimulating herbs to support effective liver function.

BURDOCK ROOT (Arctium lappa)
Blood cleanser, used for skin eruptions, dry/scaly skin conditions; digestive stimulant.

CHAPARRAL LEAF (Larrea tridentata)
Stimulates sluggish liver.

DANDELION ROOT/LEAF (Taraxacum officinale)
Blood cleanser; for inflammation and congestion of the liver and gall bladder, congestive jaundice, stimulates the flow of bile. Mild laxative, aids weight loss, lowers cholesterol and blood pressure.

FENNEL SEED (Foeniculum vulgare)
Aids digestion; relieves flatulence and colic.

MILK THISTLE SEED (Silybum marianum)
Powerful liver detoxifier, antidote for Amanita mushroom poisoning. Increases secretion and flow of bile.

OREGON GRAPE ROOT (Mahonia repens)
Liver and blood cleanser; stimulates flow of bile; anti-bacterial. Stimulates digestion and absorption. Used for sluggish liver and help alleviate hangovers.

RED CLOVER FLOWERS (Trifolium pratense)
Blood cleanser; nutritive; principal ingredient of the Hoxey cancer formula.

TOADFLAX (Linaria vulgaris) Liver cleanser; stimulates bile production; used in hepatitis, jaundice, sluggish liver. Potent—best used in small amounts in formulas.

WILD YAM ROOT (Dioscorea spp.)
Antispasmodic; carminative; anti-inflammatory; hepatic; cholagogue; diaphoretic. Used for intestinal colic, diverticulitis, painful menses, ovarian and uterine pain, rheumatoid arthritis, flatulence.

Lullaby Glycerite Formula

Children's aid to restful sleep.

ALFALFA (Medicago sativa)
Nutritive herb with high mineral and vitamin content, including Vit. K and iron.

CATNIP HERB (Nepeta cataria)
Mild sedative, soothes crankiness.

CHAMOMILE FLOWER (Matricaria recutita)
For fever and restlessness. Mild pain reliever, helps relieve colic, dispel gas. Calming.

FENNEL SEED (Foeniculum vulgare)
Aids digestion; relieves flatulence and colic; expels mucous; flavoring agent; increases digestibility of other herbs.

LEMON BALM (Melissa officinalis)
Very useful in reducing fevers during colds and flu since it induces mild perspiration. Aids digestion, reduces flatulence.

LICORICE ROOT (Glycyrrhiza glabra)
Soothing demulcent; mild laxative.

RED RASPBERRY LEAF (Rhubus idaeus)
Nutritive, relieves nausea. Remedy for childhood diarrhea.

ROSEHIPS (Rosa canina)
Nutritive, mild diuretic and laxative, mild astringent. Excellent source of vitamin C. Used for colds, flu, general debility and exhaustion, constipation.

VALERIAN ROOT (Valeriana officinalis)
Nervine, used for tension, anxiety, insomnia, emotional stress, intestinal colic, migraine headache and rheumatic pain, breaking addictions.

Lymphatic Formula

Promotes cleansing and draining of lymphatic tissue. Helps the body excrete toxic waste during infections.

BURDOCK ROOT (Arctium lappa)
Blood cleanser, used for skin eruptions, dry/scaly skin conditions; digestive stimulant.

CLEAVERS (Galium spp.)
Lymphatic tonic; alterative; diuretic. For swollen glands, cystitis, ulcers and tumors, skin disorders, painful urination.

ECHINACEA ROOT (Echinacea angustifolia)
Antiseptic; anti-microbial; anti-viral; used for sore throats, flu, colds, infections, allergies.

OCOTILLO (Fouquieria splendens)
Stimulates lymphatic drainage; improves dietary fat absorption into the lymph system. Helps drain pelvic congestion, making it useful in the treatment of hemorrhoids and varicose veins.

RED ROOT (Ceanothus americana)
Stimulates lymphatic and interstitial fluid circulation. Aids in the transport of nutrients and the elimination of waste products. Used for tonsillitis, sore throat, enlarged lymph nodes and spleen, fibrous cysts. Mild expectorant, hemostatic.

WILD INDIGO ROOT (Baptisia tinctoria)
Emetic; purgative; lymph cleanser; for focused local infection such as sore throat, laryngitis, tonsillitis, pharyngitis, gingivitis, mouth ulcers and pyorrhea, also inflamed lymph nodes. Best used in small amounts in a formula.

Male Glandular Formula

Formulated to gently balance male glandular function.
Warning—has been known to increase libido.

DAMIANA (Turnera diffusa)
Diuretic, relieves irritation of urinary mucus membranes; genito-urinary stimulant effect leading to its use as an aphrodisiac; improves digestion; laxative; tonic.

GINSENG ROOT (Panax quinquefolium)
Adaptogenic, decreases the effect of stress. Increases capillary circulation in brain; reproductive tonic; anti-depressant; equalizes blood pressure. Used for general exhaustion and weakness; aids digestion. Promotes longevity.

LICORICE ROOT (Glycyrrhiza glabra)
Specific for adrenal gland insufficiency; hormonal balance.

SAW PALMETTO (Serenoa repens)
Tones and strengthens male reproductive system, used for prostate enlargement and infection, enhances endurance.

Menopause Formula

Balancing and supportive herbs to ease transition symptoms such as mood swings, hot flashes and irregular menses associated with menopause.

ALFALFA (Medicago sativa)
Nutritive herb with high mineral and vitamin content including Vit. K and iron; estrogen precursor for menopause; mild diuretic.

BLACK COHOSH ROOT (Cimicifuga racemosa) [P/C]
Antispasmodic, relieves hot flashes in menopausal women; mild sedative.

DANDELION ROOT/LEAF (Taraxacum officinale)
Blood cleanser; powerful and safe diuretic, high in potassium. Mild laxative, aids weight loss, lowers cholesterol and blood pressure.

DONG QUAI ROOT (Angelica sinensis)
Female hormone regulator, alleviates cramping and premenstrual distress.

GINSENG ROOT (Panax quinquefolium)
Adaptogenic, decreases the effect of stress. Increases capillary circulation in brain; anti-depressant; equalizes blood pressure. Used for general exhaustion and weakness; aids digestion. Promotes longevity.

HAWTHORNE BERRY (Crataegus oxycantha)
Heart and circulatory tonic.

LICORICE ROOT (Glycyrrhiza glabra)
Specific for adrenal gland insufficiency; anti-inflammatory.

MOTHERWORT HERB (Leonurus cardiaca) [P/C]
Antispasmodic; cardiac tonic; reduces tension, anxiety.

NETTLE (Urtica dioica)
Nutritive, rich in iron, silica, and potassium. For anemia.

OAT SEED (Avena sativa)
Antispasmodic; soothes and supports nervous system; for depression, insomnia, hysteria, irritation and anxiety.

Muscle /Bruise Spray

For muscular sprains, strains and bruises. External Use Only

ARNICA FLOWER (Arnica cordifolia)
Topical use for bruises, sprains, strains and other athletic injuries, including swelling. Use on unbroken skin.

CALENDULA FLOWER (Calendula officinalis)
Anti-inflammatory; astringent. Use topically. Helps re-absorb blood from bruised tissue, relieves sprains and strains.

ST. JOHN'S WORT (Hypericum perforatum)
Extract and oil used externally for bruises, strains, sprains, contusions, wounds.

Nausea Formula

For motion sickness, indigestion, nausea.

COW PARSNIP ROOT/SEED (Heracleum lanatum)
Anti-nauseant; stimulant; hypotensive; emmenagogue; antispasmodic; carminative.

GINGER ROOT (Asarum canadense)
Used for nausea, motion sickness. Diaphoretic, helps break fevers; stimulant; carminative; aids in utilization of other herbs.

PEPPERMINT LEAF (Mentha piperita)
For upset stomach, heartburn, nausea, colds, flu, congestion, nervous headache and agitation, also diarrhea and flatulence. Adds flavor to other herbs.

Pain Formula

Anodyne and anti-spasmodic herbs which have traditionally been used for headaches and muscular pain.

BLUE VERVAIN (Verbena spp.)
Sedative, anti-depressant, causes sweating, reduces fevers, anti-spasmodic, mild analgesic.

CHAMOMILE FLOWER (Matricaria recutita)
Sedative, carminative, antispasmodic, anodyne.

FEVERFEW LEAF/FLOWER (Tanacetum parthenium)
Anti-inflammatory, used for rheumatoid arthritis, migraine headache relief (long term basis). Mild febrifuge.

GINGER ROOT (Asarum canadense)
Diaphoretic, stimulant; carminative; aids in utilization of other herbs, reduces nausea.

JAMAICAN DOGWOOD (Piscidia erythrina)
Sedative; anodyne; smooth muscle antispasmodic. For insomnia, neuralgia, menstrual cramping. Relieves coughing, reduces fevers.

PASSIONFLOWER (Passiflora incarnata)
Sedative, hypnotic, antispasmodic, anodyne. Relieves nerve pain, promotes restful sleep. Calms hysteria.

ROSEMARY LEAF (Rosmarinus officinalis)
Circulatory and nerve stimulant, used for tension headache associated with dyspepsia, also depression. Anti-bacterial; antifungal.

VALERIAN ROOT (Valeriana officinalis)
Powerful nervine, used for tension, anxiety, insomnia, emotional stress, intestinal colic, menstrual cramps, migraine headache and rheumatic pain.

WHITE WILLOW BARK (Salix alba)
Astringent, contains salicin, reduces inflammation. For headache, neuralgia, fevers, hayfever, arthritis and rheumatism.

WILD LETTUCE HERB (Lactuca spp.)
Sedative, calms restlessness and anxiety, reduces spasms.

Parasite Formula

A broad spectrum formula for intestinal parasites.

BLACK WALNUT HULLS (Juglans nigra)
Vermifuge; antifungal, for Candida, athlete's foot, ringworm, etc.; astringent, used for skin eruptions. Helps break down cystic tissue.

BUTTERNUT BARK (Juglans cineraria)
Gentle tonic, vermifuge.

CHAPARRO (Castela emoryi)
Active inhibitor of intestinal protozoa. Used to prevent and alleviate amoebic dysentery and giardia.

ECHINACEA ROOT (Echinacea angustifolia)
Stimulates immune response; antiseptic; anti-microbial; anti-viral.

GARLIC BULB/SEED (Allium sativum)
Anthelmintic, antibiotic; anti-microbial; antiseptic; antiviral. Has long, successful history in treatment of tapeworm, round worm, pinworm and other parasites. Makes internal environment totally unfavorable to their survival.

GOLDENSEAL ROOT (Hydrastis canadensis)
Antiseptic, used internally and topically for infection, sore throat, gastritis, ulceration and colitis.

MARSHMALLOW ROOT (Althaea officinalis)
Soothing demulcent, used for gastro-intestinal inflammation, buffers the other herbs in the formula.

QUASSIA (Pycrasma excelsa)
Bitter tonic and stomachic; antispasmodic; anthelmintic. Used to rid the body of parasites and improve digestion.

WORMWOOD LEAF (Artemisia absinthium)
Reduces fevers, will inhibit roundworm and pinworm infestation when used consistently for a week or two. Stimulates sweating in dry fevers. *Use small amounts in the formula, preferably with herbalist or physician supervision.*

PMS Formula

For mood swings, cramping, and general misery experienced immediately prior to the female menstrual cycle.

ALFALFA (Medicago sativa)
Nutritive herb with high mineral and vitamin content including Vit. K and iron; estrogen precursor for menopause; mild diuretic.

BLACK COHOSH ROOT (Cimicifuga racemosa) [P/C]
Antispasmodic used for menstrual cramping, coughs, muscle spasms; emmenagogue; relieves hot flashes in menopausal women; mild sedative.

BLUE VERVAIN (Verbena spp.)
Soothes cranky children, sedative, anti-depressant, diaphoretic, febrifuge, antispasmodic, mild analgesic.

CHASTE BERRY (Vitex agnus castus)
Reproductive tonic, stimulates and normalizes pituitary function. For menstrual cramps, PMS, menopause, post birth control pill rebalancing.

DONG QUAI ROOT (Angelica sinensis)
Female hormone regulator, alleviates cramping and premenstrual distress.

OAT SEED (Avena sativa)
Antispasmodic; soothes and supports nervous system; for depression, insomnia, hysteria, irritation and anxiety. Helpful in breaking addictions.

PASSIONFLOWER (Passiflora incarnata)
Sedative, antispasmodic, anodyne. Relieves nerve pain, promotes restful sleep. Has been used for seizures and hysteria.

Professor Cayenne's "TNT" Formula

This formula is different, being extracted in raw, organic apple cider vinegar instead of grain alcohol and distilled water. It is used for the early onset of colds and flu. It also makes a great medicinal salad dressing!

CAYENNE FRUIT (Capsicum frutescens)
Equalizes circulation; for cold hands and feet; strengthens heart; stimulant; carminative; styptic. Antiseptic, used as a gargle for persistent cough.

GARLIC BULB/SEED (Allium sativum)
Antibiotic; anti-microbial; antiseptic; antiviral; anthelmintic. For colds, flu, chronic bronchitis, infections, also to reduce blood pressure and cholesterol.

GINGER ROOT (Asarum canadense)
Used for nausea, motion sickness; diaphoretic, helps break fevers; stimulant; carminative; aids in utilization of other herbs.

HORSERADISH ROOT (Armoracia rusticana)
Stimulant; for flu, fevers, sinus and respiratory congestion. Sialagogue, carminative, mild laxative, diuretic.

ONION (Allium cepa)
Diuretic, expectorant, carminative, antiseptic, antispasmodic, anthelmintic. Helps alleviate putrefaction in the gastrointestinal tract. Used to alleviate cold and flu symptoms.

PARSLEY LEAF and ROOT (Petroselenum crispum) [P/C]
Diuretic, carminative, antispasmodic, emmenagogue, expectorant.

Prostate Formula

Herbal allies to strengthen and support the prostate gland.

CLEAVERS (Galium spp.)
Lymphatic tonic; alterative; diuretic. For swollen glands, cystitis, ulcers and tumors, painful urination.

COTTON ROOT (Gossypium herbaceum)
Increases tone and contractibility of seminal vesicles.

COUCHGRASS ROOT (Agropyron repens)
Demulcent; anti-microbial; antilithic; for cystitis, urethritis, prostatitis, kidney stones and gravel.

ECHINACEA ROOT (Echinacea angustifolia)
Stimulates immune response; antiseptic; anti-microbial; anti-viral; used for sore throats, flu, colds, infections, allergies.

GRAVEL ROOT (Eupatorium purpureum)
For kidney and urinary infections and stones, prostatitis, pelvic inflammatory disease; rheumatism and gout.

MARSHMALLOW ROOT (Althaea officinalis)
Soothes irritated tissue, buffers other herbs in formula.

SAW PALMETTO (Serenoa repens)
Tones and strengthens male reproductive system, used for prostate enlargement and infection, enhances endurance.

Quit Smoking Formula

Formulated to alleviate the nervousness associated with nicotine withdrawal while stimulating detoxification and expectoration.

ANISE SEED (Pimpinella anisum)
Antispasmodic and expectorant.

CHAMOMILE FLOWER (Matricaria recutita)
Sedative, carminative, antispasmodic, anodyne.

DANDELION ROOT/LEAF (Taraxacum officinale)
Blood cleanser; powerful and safe diuretic, high in potassium; cholagogue, for inflammation and congestion of the liver and gall bladder, congestive jaundice. Mild laxative, aids weight loss, lowers cholesterol and blood pressure.

GRINDELIA BUDS/FLOWERS (Grindelia spp.)
Expectorant; anti-spasmodic; for bronchitis, sinus congestion, bladder infections; topically for poison oak and ivy, insect bites.

LICORICE ROOT (Glycyrrhiza glabra)
Specific for adrenal gland insufficiency; demulcent; expectorant for coughs and respiratory congestion; anti-inflammatory; laxative.

LOBELIA HERB (Lobelia inflata)
Respiratory stimulant; anti-asthmatic; anti-emetic (small dose), emetic (large dose). Used for bronchitis and bronchitic asthma, whooping cough, muscular cramping and pain.

OAT SEED (Avena sativa)
Antispasmodic; soothes and supports nervous system; for depression, insomnia, hysteria, irritation and anxiety. Helpful in decreasing the irritability associated with nicotine withdrawal.

VALERIAN ROOT (Valeriana officinalis)
Powerful nervine, used for tension, anxiety, insomnia, emotional stress, intestinal colic, menstrual cramps, migraine headache and rheumatic pain, breaking addictions.

Reishi/Shiitake Formula

Adaptogenic, immune stimulating formula. Supports nerve and metabolic function during high stress periods. Especially good for people who constantly out-flow energy without enough in-flow (also known as Type A personalities).

REISHI MUSHROOM (Ganoderma lucidum)

Adaptogenic, used to alleviate the effects of stress. Strengthens heart, protects liver, soothes nerves. Normalizes blood pressure. Inhibits the release of histamine, thus relieving the allergic inflammatory response. Supports adrenal function. Stimulates the immune system. Slows the aging process. Anti-carcinogenic. Anti-bacterial.

SHIITAKE MUSHROOM (Lentinus edodes)

Adaptogenic. Increases the production of interferon, thus reducing the possibility of tumor development. Anti-viral. Helps the body excrete excess cholesterol.

Rejuvenation Formula

A true tonic formula for physical and mental longevity.

ALFALFA (Medicago sativa)
Nutritive herb with high mineral and vitamin content including Vit. K and iron; mild diuretic.

GINKGO LEAF (Ginkgo biloba)
Stimulates cerebral circulation and oxygenation, mental clarity and alertness, improves memory. Used to prevent strokes.

GINSENG ROOT (Panax quinquefolium)
Adaptogenic, decreases the effect of stress. Increases capillary circulation in brain; reproductive tonic; anti-depressant; equalizes blood pressure. Used for general exhaustion and weakness; aids digestion. Promotes longevity.

GOTU KOLA LEAF (Centella asiatica)
Used to increase mental stamina, alleviate depression and anxiety, improve memory and promote longevity. Increases energy and endurance.

LICORICE ROOT (Glycyrrhiza glabra)
Specific for adrenal gland insufficiency; demulcent; expectorant for coughs and respiratory congestion; anti-inflammatory; laxative.

OAT SEED (Avena sativa)
Antispasmodic; soothes and supports nervous system; for depression, insomnia, hysteria, irritation and anxiety. Helpful in breaking addictions.

Restful Sleep Formula

For those whose brains will not shut off at night. For the agitation generated by too much mental activity and too little physical activity. Insomnia and nervous tension. Helps promote sleep when changing time zones while traveling.

CATNIP HERB (Nepeta cataria)
Calming, soothing, gently tranquilizing. Carminative, diaphoretic, antispasmodic, mild febrifuge. For indigestion, flatulence and colic; mild astringent, specific for childhood fevers and diarrhea.

CHAMOMILE FLOWER (Matricaria recutita)
Sedative, carminative, antispasmodic, anodyne. Children's herb, especially for fever and restlessness.

HOPS STROBILE (Humulus lupus)
Sedative; hypnotic. Used for anxiety, tension, insomnia. Reduces nervous irritability, promotes restful sleep.

PASSIONFLOWER (Passiflora incarnata)
Sedative, hypnotic, antispasmodic, anodyne. Relieves nerve pain, promotes restful sleep. Has been used for seizures and hysteria.

SKULLCAP HERB (Scutellaria lateriflora)
Nervine; sedative; antispasmodic; used for nervous tension, hysteria, epileptic seizures, withdrawal from substance abuse and the irritability of PMS.

VALERIAN ROOT (Valeriana officinalis)
Powerful nervine, used for tension, anxiety, insomnia, emotional stress, intestinal colic, menstrual cramps, migraine headache and rheumatic pain.

Stress Formula

A gently balancing, nerve supportive formula for high stress periods.

BLUE VERVAIN (Verbena spp.)
Soothes crankiness, sedative, anti-depressant, diaphoretic, febrifuge, antispasmodic, mild analgesic.

CHAMOMILE FLOWER (Matricaria recutita)
Sedative, carminative, antispasmodic, anodyne. Used for fever and restlessness.

GINSENG ROOT (Panax quinquefolium)
Adaptogenic, decreases the effect of stress. Increases capillary circulation in brain; reproductive tonic; anti-depressant; equalizes blood pressure. Used for general exhaustion, hysteria, irritation and anxiety. Helpful in breaking addictions. Alleviates exhaustion and weakness; aids digestion. Promotes longevity.

OAT SEED (Avena sativa)
Antispasmodic; soothes and supports nervous system; for depression, insomnia, hysteria, irritation and anxiety. Helpful in breaking addictions.

PASSIONFLOWER (Passiflora incarnata)
Sedative, hypnotic, antispasmodic, anodyne. Relieves nerve pain, promotes restful sleep. Calms hysteria.

PRODIGIOSA (Brickellia grandiflora)
Helps regulate *overuse* of fight or flight response by moderating epinephrine's stimulation of liver to break down stored glycogen into blood sugar.

SKULLCAP HERB (Scutellaria lateriflora)
Nervine; sedative; antispasmodic; used for nervous tension, hysteria, epileptic seizures, withdrawal from substance abuse and the irritability of PMS.

ST. JOHN'S WORT (Hypericum perforatum)
Used internally as an immune system stimulant; for retro-viral infections; expectorant; anti-bacterial, speeds wound and burn healing; antidepressant; used to treat bedwetting and children's nightmares.

Throat Extract/Spray Formula

For sore, scratchy, irritated and inflamed throats. Works very well in conjunction with Vitamin C supplementation. Can be sprayed directly into the throat, taken internally or used as a gargle.

CAYENNE FRUIT (Capsicum frutescens)
Circulatory stimulant. Antiseptic, used as gargle for sore throat, persistent cough, laryngitis.

ECHINACEA ROOT (Echinacea angustifolia)
Stimulates immune system; facilitates lymphatic drainage, antiseptic; anti-microbial; anti-viral; used for sore throats, flu, colds, infections, allergies.

GOLDENSEAL ROOT (Hydrastis canadensis)
Antiseptic, used internally and topically for infection, sore throat.

LICORICE ROOT (Glycyrrhiza glabra)
Soothing demulcent; expectorant for coughs and respiratory congestion; anti-inflammatory; laxative.

MYRRH GUM (Commiphora myrrha)
Antiseptic; anti-microbial; astringent. Used for mouth ulcers, sore throat, gingivitis, pyorrhea, sinusitis and pharyngitis.

OSHA' ROOT (Ligusticum porterii)
Strong antiviral, used for herpes, sore throat, colds, flu; bronchial expectorant; immune stimulating properties.

PROPOLIS
Antiseptic, antibacterial. Waxy nature makes it useful for coating and isolating areas of throat inflammation to prevent spread of infection, and to bind the other herbs to the throat for longer lasting effect.

USNEA LICHEN (Usnea spp.)
Strong antibiotic, very effective for strep throat; antiviral; for internal infections, staph, trichomonas, etc., infected wounds.

Vaginitis Formula

An antiseptic, antibiotic formula which assists the body in healing vaginal infections and irritations. Bitter taste, best mixed with juice or tea.

ECHINACEA ROOT (Echinacea angustifolia)
Immune stimulant; antiseptic; anti-microbial; anti-viral; used for sore throats, flu, colds, infections.

GARLIC BULB/SEED (Allium sativum)
Antibiotic; anti-microbial; antiseptic; antiviral. Drives infection from the body.

GOLDENSEAL ROOT (Hydrastis canadensis)
Antiseptic, used internally and topically for infection, sore throat, gastritis, ulceration and colitis. Infusion of the fresh or dried root used as douche for vaginitis.

OSHA' ROOT (Ligusticum porterii)
Strong antiviral, used for herpes, sore throat, colds, flu; bronchial expectorant; immune stimulating properties.

PEPPERMINT LEAF (Mentha piperita)
For upset stomach, heartburn, nausea, colds, flu, congestion, nervous headache and agitation, also diarrhea and flatulence. Adds flavor to the formula.

RED ROOT (Ceanothus americana)
Lymphatic stimulant, facilitating the excretion of metabolic toxins from the body. Used for infections, enlarged lymph nodes and spleen, fibrous cysts.

USNEA LICHEN (Usnea spp.)
Strong antibiotic; antiviral; antifungal; for internal infections, strep, staph, trichomonas, etc., infected wounds. Also used for pneumonia, TB and Lupus.

Vein Toning Formula

Supports and strengthens vascular integrity.

BLUE VERVAIN (Verbena spp.)
Tonic, diaphoretic, mild analgesic.

DANDELION ROOT/LEAF (Taraxacum officinale)
Blood cleanser; powerful and safe diuretic, high in potassium; cholagogue, for inflammation and congestion of the liver and gall bladder, congestive jaundice. Mild laxative, aids weight loss, lowers cholesterol and blood pressure.

HAWTHORNE BERRY (Crataegus oxycantha)
Heart and circulatory tonic.

MELILOT (Melilotus officinalis)
Spasmolytic. Reduces blood stagnation.

MILK THISTLE SEED (Silybum marianum)
Powerful liver detoxifier.

OCOTILLO (Fouquieria splendens)
Reduces pelvic congestion and pressure on the pelvic veins.

SHEPHERD'S PURSE (Capsella Bursa-pastoris)
Hemostatic; astringent; diuretic.

STONE ROOT (Collinsonia canadensis)
Strengthens structural integrity of veins, used for varicose veins, hemorrhoids, anal fissures, and rectal spasms.

SYRUPS

Syrups are a tasty, soothing way to ingest herbs. They are traditionally made with a sweet tasting base such as honey or glycerin. Honey has antiseptic properties. The following syrups are wonderful allies to have around during the cold season.

Cough Formula Syrup

Soothing, antispasmodic herbs in a honey glycerin base to calm coughing.

BLUE VERVAIN (Verbena spp.)
Sedative; antispasmodic; diaphoretic, promotes mild sweating to excrete toxins and decrease fever; mild pain reliever.

CAYENNE FRUIT (Capsicum frutescens)
Antiseptic, stimulates circulation to help metabolize nutrients and excrete toxins.

COLTSFOOT (Tussilago farfara)
Soothing expectorant, demulcent, antispasmodic, astringent, anti-inflammatory. For irritating coughs, bronchitis, asthma laryngitis, throat catarrh.

ELECAMPANE ROOT (Inula helenium)
Expectorant; diaphoretic; anti-bacterial; anti-tussive; stomachic; for irritating bronchial coughs, bronchitis, emphysema, asthma and bronchitic asthma.

JAMAICAN DOGWOOD (Piscidia erythrina)
Sedative; pain reliever; smooth muscle antispasmodic. Relieves coughing, reduces fevers.

LICORICE ROOT (Glycyrrhiza glabra)
Soothing demulcent; expectorant for coughs and respiratory congestion; anti-inflammatory; laxative.

LOBELIA HERB (Lobelia inflata)
Respiratory stimulant; anti-asthmatic. Used for bronchitis and bronchitic asthma, whooping cough, muscular cramping and pain.

Expectorant Formula Syrup

Herbs which promote the expectoration of excess mucus from the respiratory system. Honey/glycerin base.

BONESET (Eupatorium perfoliatum)
For flu symptoms, aches and pains; clears mucus congestion; reduces fevers; muscular rheumatism.

COLTSFOOT (Tussilago farfara)
Soothing expectorant, demulcent, antispasmodic, astringent, anti-inflammatory. For irritating coughs, bronchitis, asthma, laryngitis, throat catarrh.

GRINDELIA BUDS/FLOWERS (Grindelia spp.)
Expectorant; anti-spasmodic; for bronchitis, mucus congestion.

HOREHOUND HERB (Marrubium vulgare)
Effective decongestant, expectorant.

HYSSOP LEAF (Hyssopus officinalis)
Anti-spasmodic; nervine; expectorant; diaphoretic, sedative, carminative. For chronic congestion.

LICORICE ROOT (Glycyrrhiza glabra)
Soothing demulcent; expectorant for coughs and respiratory congestion; anti-inflammatory; laxative.

MULLEIN LEAF (Verbascum thapsus)
Expectorant; demulcent; reduces respiratory inflammation.

OSHA' ROOT (Ligusticum porterii)
Bronchial expectorant, strong antiviral, used for sore throat, colds, flu; stimulates immune system.

Garlic Formula Syrup

GARLIC SYRUP?!? Believe it or not, it's really tasty. Also known as an oxymel, this formula is made with fresh garlic bulbs, raw, organic apple cider vinegar and raw honey. The vinegar neutralizes the odor and taste of the garlic. Once you experience how well this works, you'll make it a part of your standard home herbal remedy chest.

GARLIC BULB/SEED (Allium sativum)
Used primarily for its antibiotic effect.

Throat Soothing Syrup

In a base of honey and glycerin, this syrup is wonderful for sore throats and is also useful for laryngitis.

BALM OF GILEAD (Populus gileadensis)
Soothes, disinfects and astringes mucous membranes. Specific for laryngitis, coughs and sore throat.

COLTSFOOT (Tussilago farfara)
Soothing expectorant, demulcent, antispasmodic, astringent, anti-inflammatory. For irritating coughs, bronchitis, asthma laryngitis, throat catarrh.

ECHINACEA ROOT (Echinacea angustifolia)
Powerful immune stimulant; antiseptic; anti-microbial; anti-viral; used for sore throats, flu, colds, infections.

PROPOLIS
Antiseptic, antibacterial. Waxy nature makes it useful for coating and isolating areas of throat inflammation to prevent spread of infection and to bind the other ingredients to the throat for longer lasting effect.

SLIPPERY ELM (Ulmus rhubra)
Nutritive, reduces inflammation, soothes mucus membranes.

SALVES/BALMS

Salves are useful as topical healing agents. For wounds, they should generally be used as a skin dressing after a scab has formed. Otherwise, the body might retain bacteria underneath, leading to infection. Wash the wound and apply an antiseptic first. Salves and balms work particularly well on bruises, sprains, strains and to otherwise decongest tissue.

Bruise Salve

ARNICA FLOWER (Arnica Cordifolia)
External Use Only. Topical use for bruises, sprains, strains and other athletic injuries, including swelling. Use on unbroken skin.

CALENDULA FLOWER (Calendula officinalis)
Anti-inflammatory; astringent; styptic; antifungal. Use topically for wounds, ulcers, burns, abscesses.

ST. JOHN'S WORT (Hypericum perforatum)
Used externally for bruises, strains, sprains, contusions, wounds. Speeds wound and burn healing.

Bug Repelling Salve

To discourage insects from trespassing on your body. The following essential oils are all known for their insect repellant properties. Carried in a base of olive oil and beeswax.

CITRONELLA (Ceylonese or Javanese)

EUCALYPTUS (Eucalyptus citriodora)

LAVENDER (Lavandula officinalis)

PENNYROYAL (Mentha pelugium)

Muscle Easing Salve

In a base of olive oil and beeswax. A deep heating rub for muscle tension, soreness, sprains and strains.

ARNICA FLOWER (Arnica cordifolia)
External Use Only. Topical use for bruises, sprains, strains and other athletic injuries, including swelling. Use on unbroken skin.

CAJEPUT (Melaleuca leucadendron)
Analgesic (pain relieving).

CAMPHOR (Cinnamomum camphora)
Analgesic, antispasmodic, anti-neuralgic, anti-rheumatic.

CAYENNE FRUIT (Capsicum frutescens)
Stimulates circulation, reduces tissue congestion. Creates heat.

MENTHOL (Mentha arvensis) Isolate
Cooling, anti-inflammatory, analgesic.

ST. JOHN'S WORT (Hypericum perforatum)
Oil used externally for bruises, strains, sprains, contusions, wounds.

WINTERGREEN (Methyl salycilate) Derivative
Analgesic.

Skin Soothing Salve

A soothing blend of skin healing herbs in an olive oil and beeswax base.

CALENDULA FLOWER (Calendula officinalis)
Anti-inflammatory; astringent; styptic; antifungal; topically for wounds, ulcers, burns, abscesses.

CAYENNE FRUIT (Capsicum frutescens)
Stimulates circulation, reduces tissue congestion. Creates heat.

CHICKWEED HERB (Stellaria media)
Restorative; soothing demulcent.

COMFREY ROOT/LEAF (Symphytum officinalis)
External Use. Speeds healing of sprains, strains, fractures and surface wounds.

GOLDENSEAL ROOT (Hydrastis canadensis)
Antiseptic, used topically for infection.

MALLOW (Malva rotundifolia)
Astringent, demulcent, emollient, anti-inflammatory; speeds healing.

PLANTAIN LEAF (Plantago spp.)
Astringent; used for external wounds and sores, insect bites.

ST. JOHN'S WORT (Hypericum perforatum)
Used externally for bruises, strains, sprains, contusions, wounds. Anti-bacterial, speeds wound and burn healing.

Vapor Decongestant Salve

Herbal sister to Vick's Vapor Rub, using olive oil and beeswax instead of petroleum. Use as a decongestant rub, in steam vaporizers or smear on a tissue and inhale to decongest sinuses.

CAMPHOR (Cinnamomum camphora)
Analgesic, antispasmodic, anti-neuralgic, anti-rheumatic.

CLOVE (Eugenia caryophyllata)
Stimulating antiseptic.

LAVENDER (Lavandula officinalis)
Antiseptic, decongestant, calming, antispasmodic.

MENTHOL (Mentha arvensis) Isolate
Cooling, anti-inflammatory, analgesic.

PEPPERMINT (Mentha piperita)
Cooling, decongesting, pain relieving.

ST. JOHN'S WORT (Hypericum perforatum)
Oil used externally for bruises, strains, sprains, contusions, wounds.

WINTERGREEN (Methyl salycilate) Derivative
Cooling, fragrant analgesic.

Ear Oil Formula

A soothing, antiseptic, antibiotic oil which is phenomenally effective in the treatment of both acute and chronic ear infections.
Contra-indicated in cases of eardrum perforation.

CALENDULA FLOWER (Calendula officinalis)
Anti-inflammatory; astringent; antifungal.

GARLIC BULB/SEED (Allium sativum)
Antibiotic; anti-microbial; antiseptic; antiviral.

MULLEIN LEAF (Verbascum thapsus)
Anti-inflammatory, soothing.

ST. JOHN'S WORT (Hypericum perforatum)
Soothing, healing, activates immune response.

Common Problems/ Natural Remedies

This list is compiled for educational purposes. The remedies are suggestions only and are not intended as a substitute for professional assistance when needed.

Emergency First Aid

Breathing, bleeding and shock are the first priorities in emergency first aid situations. Stay calm and analyze the situation, then assist. (You can take a homeopathic flower remedy here.)

Breathing: Take a class in CPR (Cardio-Pulmonary Resuscitation) at your local Red Cross. It's worth it!

Bleeding: Direct pressure on the wound helps stop the blood flow, as do styptic herbs such as Yarrow and Horsetail. Make sure the wound has been thoroughly flushed with blood, soap and water or an antiseptic solution before you encourage it to close and heal, otherwise, you will seal the bacteria inside and risk infection.

Shock: Keep the patient warm and elevate their legs. Flower essence remedies such as *Rescue Remedy*™ or *Flowers formula* are helpful to keep the person (and you) calm and level headed. The Essential Rescue aromatherapy inhaler is also useful. Do not give fluids to someone who is in shock.

Abrasions: Wash well, then apply an antiseptic spray or skin soothing salve. Bandage if necessary.

Abscesses: Infection Formula, Lymph Formula, Detox Formula, vitamin C. Eat plenty of Garlic and drink distilled water.

Acne: Healthy Skin Formula (internally and externally), Detox Formula, Liver Formula. External—vapor steam of Lemon, Lavender, Geranium and Chamomile essential oils; fresh application of Aloe vera.

Air Sickness: See *Motion Sickness.*

Anemia: Iron Formula, eat plenty of dark leafy greens.

Anxiety: Stress Formula, Adrenal Formula, Children's Calming Glycerite Formula, Essential Tranquility or Balance aromatherapy inhalers. Dietary calcium and B complex.

Arthritis: Joint Formula.

Asthma: Asthma Formula, Bronchial Formula, Stress Formula. (Please dissipate alcohol before using.)

Athlete's Foot: See *Fungal Infections.*

Bee Sting: Infection Formula, Antiseptic Spray Formula, Plantain, Comfrey or Clay Poultices; Papain powder, Honey.

Bladder Infections: Kidney Formula, Infection Formula, Cranberry juice or extract; plenty of vitamin C.

Bloody Nose: Apply pressure on either side of the nose. Apply cold compresses to the sinuses. Dampen a piece of gauze with water, dip it into powdered Yarrow or Horsetail and insert into nostril. Apply strong pressure with your fingernail to the outside corner of the base of the little "pinky" fingernail which is on the same side as the nostril which is bleeding.

Bronchitis: Onion Poultice, Infection Formula, Bronchial Formula, Expectorant Formula, Expectorant Syrup, Ginger Fomentation, Vapor Steam; plenty of Vitamin C.

Bruises: Muscle/Bruise Liniment Formula, Bruise Salve, fresh Comfrey Leaf Poultice.

Burns (minor): FIRST immerse the burned area in ice cold water or apply ice, then treat with one of the following: fresh Aloe Vera leaf, Burn Spray Formula, Dr. Christopher's Burn Ointment (see Natural Therapies section), or vitamin E.

Chapped Lips and Skin: Skin Soothing Salve.

Chiggers: Bug Salve or Spray, Echinacea extract, Infection Formula.

Cold Sores: Osha' Root extract or Infection Formula applied externally; Antiviral Formula internally. Supplement with non-acidic vitamin C, Acidophilus and Garlic (antibiotic).

Colds/Flu: Onion Horseradish Vinegar Formula, Infection Formula, Antiviral Formula, Immune Formula, Echinacea extract, Immune Formula, Miso soup, Peppermint tea, distilled water, Laxative Formula if constipated, Pain Formula for aches and pain, and plenty of REST!

Colic: Children's Calming Glycerite Formula, Digestive Formula; Peppermint or mild Ginger tea.

Computer Stress Syndrome: Computer Stress Formula, Stress Formula, Rejuvenation Formula, Adrenal Formula; supplement with B vitamins, sea vegetables in diet. Grow Spider plants in your office to decrease ambient radiation.

Constipation: Laxative formula; drink more water! Eat more fresh fruits and vegetables and more dietary fiber in the form of whole grains, psyllium and flax seed. Eat less meat. Drink 2 tsp.

sea salt in 1 qt. warm water on an empty stomach upon arising in the morning. Do not eat until the bowel has evacuated. Warm water enema.

Coughing: You can make a cough syrup from the Infection Formula (or any appropriate herbal extract for that matter), simply by adding honey or glycerin. Try Expectorant Formula, Cough Formula, Bronchial Formula, Cough Syrup, Garlic Syrup.

Cradle Cap: Brush the scalp gently in a circular motion with a wet baby brush dipped in shampoo. Rinse out the scales as you loosen them. Supplement the diet with Oatstraw, Nettle, Chamomile, Alfalfa or Horsetail tea.

Cramps: Menstrual or muscular, try Cramp Formula, Ginger Fomentation and/or Castor Oil pack. Add dietary calcium.

Cuts: See *Wounds.*

Dandruff: Healthy Skin Formula, supplement with essential fatty acids, B vitamins, Acidophilus, Sea vegetables.

Depression: Essential Joy aromatherapy inhaler, St. John's Wort extract, Stress Formula, PMS Formula, Menopause Formula, Rejuvenation Formula; supplement with B-Complex vitamins.

Diarrhea: As with vomiting, let the body do its work first, and only if the person becomes weak or dehydrated should you stop the process. *Do* supplement with fluids and electrolytes. Potassium rich, potato peeling broth is helpful—wash an organic potato and cut thickly into the skin, forming peels 1/2" thick. Put into distilled water if available, simmer for 20 minutes covered, and drink. Miso soup is also good. Try Digestive Formula to increase digestion. Black Cherry juice (high in iron) is helpful, also Red Raspberry leaf tea.

Dysentery: Parasite Formula, Detox Formula, Liver Formula; Get professional diagnosis and assistance.

Earaches: Mullein-Garlic Oil. Warm oil, put 4-5 drops in ear, stuff with cotton. Onion Poultice or Castor Oil pack. (Caution: Not to be used in cases of eardrum perforation!)

Eczema: Eczema Formula, Healthy Skin Formula; essential fatty acid supplementation.

Eye Infections: Clear Eyes Formula, Eyewash Kit (see instructions in Therapies section). Infection Formula.

Fatigue: Iron Formula, Rejuvenation Formula, Adrenal Formula, Computer Stress Formula; supplement with B-Complex. Rest!

Fevers: First give the fever a chance to do its work. Give plenty of fluids such as Peppermint tea & distilled water. Each fever is different, pay attention and watch its pattern. Over 102° indicates need for professional consultation. Try Pain Formula, Infection Formula, Elder/Peppermint/Yarrow tea (equal parts), Ginger baths.

Fingernail Problems: Healthy Skin Formula; Horsetail extract. Supplement with B-Complex.

Flatulence: Use Digestive Formula immediately after meals. Better food combining. Better preparation procedure in cooking beans (soak overnight, add Apple Cider Vinegar, Savory). Digestive enzymes.

Fleas: Bug Formula Spray or Salve; supplement with Garlic, B-Complex.

Fluid Retention: Diuretic Formula, PMS Formula. Dandelion extract.

Foreign Particle in Eye: Place a Q-Tip on top of the eyelid. Hold it there while you gently grasp the eyelashes and roll the eyelid inside out over the Q-Tip. This should allow you to see and retrieve any foreign particles with another Q-Tip. Put a chia or flax seed in corner of eye. Mucilage formed by the moistened seed will carry out foreign particle. Use Eyewash kit.

Fungal Infections: For athletes foot, jock itch, ringworm, etc. Use Anti-Fungal Spray Formula on affected area. (Be careful, it *will* stain clothing.) For ringworm, soak a small piece of cotton with the formula and tape on. Re-apply fresh solution at least twice daily. Internal fungal infections such as candidiasis, use 1 dropperful Anti-Fungal Formula 3 times daily. Get a good book on Candida and incorporate its dietary guidelines.

Gas: See *Flatulence*.

Giardia: Parasite Formula (Get professional diagnostic assistance); eat plenty of Garlic.

Gum Problems: Dental poultice packs, Tooth care kit, Fresh Breath Gum Tonic; supplement with vitamin C.

Halitosis: Fresh Breath Gum Tonic; Digestive Formula; supplement with Chlorophyll. Have dental examination for tooth decay. Colon cleansing program.

Headaches: They appear for different reasons and need to be treated differently. Try Pain Formula, Ginger Fomentation to abdomen, Digestive Formula, Laxative Formula, or chiropractic adjustment. Document when they happen and what your lifestyle was like immediately preceding the onset. Check diet, constipation, fluid intake, exposure to environmental toxins, stress level, etc. For chronic headaches, half the battle is identifying what triggers it and avoiding that stimulus.

Hemorrhoids: Fresh Aloe suppositories (see "Aloe" in Natural Therapies section). There are many other natural remedies, see book list for other resources.

Herpes: Add dietary lysine (blue corn is rich in lysine and will help strengthen the body's ability to fight the virus); apply Infection Formula internally and directly to lesion, several of the herbs in it are anti-viral.

Hiccups: Take a deep breath and drink water until you burp. Try Digestive Formula or a small amount of Pain Formula for their anti-spasmodic and carminative herbs.

Hives: Stress Formula; Allergy Formula, Nettle extract, (Make sure to dissipate alcohol); supplement with B-Complex, Calcium, vitamin A.

Hot Flashes: Female Glandular Formula, Black Cohosh root extract.

Hyper/Hypo Thyroid: Sea Vegetables, Computer Stress Formula.

Indigestion: Digestive Formula, Peppermint tea or extract.

Infections, swollen glands: Infection Formula, Immune Formula, Lymph Formula, Echinacea extract, Horseradish Onion Formula, Eat raw Garlic or Garlic chives. Onion Poultice, Ginger Fomentation, Castor Oil pack. Rest!

Insect Bites: Infection Formula, Antiseptic Spray Formula, Plantain, Comfrey or Clay poultices; Papain powder; Vinegar; a dab of Muscle or Bruise salve.

Insomnia: Sleep Formula; Calcium supplements 1/2 hour before bedtime (also useful to help prevent night-time leg cramps in pregnant women).

Itching: Itch Spray Formula, Allergy Formula.

Jet Lag: Essential Rescue or Essential Balance aromatherapy inhaler; Rejuvenation Formula (Sleep Formula helps when normal sleep time is altered.)

Laryngitis: Infection Formula, Throat Extract/Spray Formula, Vapor steam, Castor Oil Pack on neck.

Libido, Lack of: Female or Male Glandular Formulas, Rejuvenation Formula, Chaste Berry extract, Essential Aphrodisiac aromatherapy inhaler.

Liver Congestion: Liver Formula, Detox Formula.

Lung Congestion: Expectorant Extract and Syrup Formulas, Bronchial Formula. Drink plenty of water, avoid dairy products. Vapor steam with vapor salve or essential oil of Eucalyptus or Sage in hot water.

Lymphatic Congestion: Lymph Formula.

Mastitis: Infection Formula, Lymph Formula; poultice of moistened, powdered or freshly ground Marshmallow root. Drink plenty of fluid; if lactating, continue nursing.

Memory, Poor: Clear Thought Formula, Essential Memory or Basil aromatherapy inhalers.

Menopause: Menopause Formula.

Menstrual Cramps: See *Cramps*.

Migraine: See *Headache*.

Morning Sickness: See *Nausea*. A chiropractic therapy is to close the ileocecal valve through external pressure manipulation. Ginger tea (sometimes contraindicated in pregnancy, although it saved me during my two!)

Motion Sickness: Nausea Formula, Ginger extract or plain Peppermint tea. Essential Rescue or Clary Sage aromatherapy inhaler.

Mumps: Antiviral Formula, Lymph Formula, Immune Formula; plenty of liquid, and vitamin C.

Muscle Aches: Muscle Liniment Spray Formula, Muscle salve, Arnica or St. John's Wort extract.

Muscle Cramps: See *Cramps*.

Nausea: Nausea Formula, Digestive Formula, Ginger extract or Peppermint tea.

Nervousness: Stress Formula, Calming Children's Glycerite Formula, Valerian Root extract; Essential Tranquility or Balance aromatherapy inhaler; supplement with B-Complex, essential fatty acids, calcium.

Nipples, cracked: Skin Soothing Salve; supplement diet with essential fatty acids.

Pain: As obtuse as "headache." Try Pain Formula; supplement with calcium.

Parasites: Parasite Formula. Eat lots of Garlic and Pumpkin seeds. Giardia and amoebic infestation require special help. See a wholistic practitioner.

PMS: PMS Formula.

Poison Ivy: Itch Spray Formula. See *Dermatitis*.

Ringworm: See *Fungal Infections*.

Scabies: Try Tea Tree oil soap. Bug Spray Formula. Ayurvedic medicine has some promising therapies; study.

Sinus Congestion: Professor Cayenne's Formula; Decongestant Heat Lamp Therapy (see Therapies); Vapor steam, inhale Vapor salve, salt water flush; sniff fresh Horseradish (deeply!), Essential Breath aromatherapy inhaler. Increase fluids, avoid dairy products.

Skin Rashes/Diaper Rash: Clay Poultice, Skin Soothing Salve, Chamomile or Calendula tea wash.

Smashed Fingers/Toes: Muscle Liniment Spray, Muscle/Bruise Salve, Arnica or St. John's Wort extract.

Smoking Addiction: Smoking Formula; Stress Formula, Detox Formula, Expectorant Formula. Essential Freedom aromatherapy inhaler. Supplement with B Complex and vitamin C.

Splinters and other small foreign objects (i.e. glass): If you can't get it out with tweezers, try a Plantain or Clay Poultice. Pine tar is helpful in cases where lots of small splinters are clustered in the skin. Smear it on. Splinters will pull out as you pull it off. Make sure you put some Antiseptic Formula on after you are finished.

Sprains/Swelling: Ice; Muscle/Bruise Salve or Liniment Spray; fresh Comfrey leaf Poultice, Arnica or St. John's Wort extract.

Sore Throat: Squirt Throat Extract/ Spray back into the throat; Slippery Elm Lozenges; Onion Poultice, Ginger Fomentation.

Stings: From ocean critters such as Portuguese Man O' War and jellyfish—First, urinate on the affected area; the ammonia in the urine will immediately relieve the sting. Then use a soothing mucilaginous herb like Comfrey Root or Slippery Elm to soothe and heal the area. (You can crush a Slippery Elm lozenge in an emergency.)

Stress: Stress Formula, Computer Stress Formula, Adrenal Formula, Reishi/Shiitake Formula; Essential Tranquility or Essential Rescue aromatherapy inhalers.

Styes: Herbal eyewash kit, Clear Eyes Formula, Infection Formula; vitamin C.

Sunburn: Aloe Burn Spray Formula, Dr. Christopher's Burn Ointment (see Therapies section), fresh Aloe vera.

Tapeworms: See *Parasites*.

Teething Pain: Pain Formula, Osha' extract rubbed on the gum. Children's Calming Glycerite Formula.

Tension: See *Stress*.

Thrush: Swab mouth with Antifungal Formula or use Antifungal Spray (stronger, contains Tea Tree oil).

Ticks: Hold incense near back of its body; tick will usually back out to get away from heat. Use Antiseptic Spray afterwards.

Toothache: Dental Poultice Pack, follow directions on pack; Cotton soaked with Osha' Root or Clove Oil.

Ulcers: Slippery Elm (make a paste with Slippery Elm powder and eat it; it will help coat the stomach and relieve pain. Cayenne (one or two capsules, twice per day). There are many other natural therapies; consult the reference section and study.

Urinary Tract Infections: See *Bladder infections*.

Vaginal infections: Goldenseal (antiseptic), Slippery Elm (to soothe), Tea Tree Oil (in a pessary form to disinfect and slow fungal infections. Goldenseal powder can be used alone to make a douche). Buy some *plain* yogurt or use acidophilus capsules. A total program for vaginal infections is as follows: First use a Goldenseal douche, then insert a pessary (herbs in a cocoa butter base molded into a bullet shape—best to use are Goldenseal and Marshmallow). Be sure to wear a pad to prevent staining; leave it in overnight. Douche again with Goldenseal in the morning, and if the infection is advanced, insert another pessary for the balance of the day. In the evening, douche with Goldenseal, then insert *plain* yogurt or acidophilus capsule and leave in through the night. Alternate the douche and yogurt implant in this manner until the infection is gone. In the meantime, increase vitamin C, use a balanced vitamin supplement. Also try Vaginitis Formula.

Varicose Veins: Vein Formula; relieve pelvic congestion with Laxative Formula, PMS Formula, Diuretic Formula, Ocotillo extract. Supplement with vitamin C.

Viral Infections: Antiviral Formula, Osha' Root extract; supplement with vitamin C.

Vomiting: To induce: Lobelia extract (10-60 drops, depending entirely on the person's reaction to it and the amount of food in the stomach; rest assured, the body will tell you when it has had enough); Syrup of Ipecac.

Vomiting: To stop:1-3 drops of Lobelia extract. (Keep in mind that the body is trying to rid itself of something it doesn't want, and respect its innate intelligence in purging itself.) Raspberry or Ginger extracts will soothe the digestive system, Nettle extract will help replenish lost nutrients. Potato peeling broth and electrolyte replacement is a good idea if the patient can keep them down.

Warts: Topical: Banana Peel Poultice, Therapies section, Cedar oil; apply Apple Cider Vinegar then follow with fresh Milkweed juice. Antiviral Formula internally and externally.

Worms: See *Parasites.*

Wounds: Encourage intial bleeding, cleanse well, then spray with antiseptic formula. Use salves only after the wound has scabbed over, otherwise you could seal over the wound before it has had time to discharge all the harmful bacteria.

Yeast Infections: See *Vaginal infections, Fungal infections.*

Natural Therapies

The value of the skills learned in this section will be apparent in lower medical bills as well as a greater sense of personal power in your own health care. A stuffy nose or a fever is manageable without a trip to the pharmacy, and athlete's foot is controllable without harsh chemicals. If you are a visually oriented learner, these therapies are shown step by step in my video, *Herbal Preparations and Natural Therapies—Creating and Using a Home Herbal Medicine Chest.*

Poultices: A poultice is the application of plant materials (or clay) to the skin. It can be made from either fresh or dried herbs. Poultices are used to soothe, heal, regenerate tissue, stimulate circulation and organ function, warm and relax muscles, and draw out toxins or foreign particles.

Simple Plantain Poultice

Plantain is one of many wayside plants that is an invaluable first aid for cuts, scrapes, bee stings and burns. It is called Nature's bandaid with good reason, having also the distinct advantage of being found nearly everywhere. It is well known for its ability to draw out glass and other objects which get deeply imbedded in the skin as well as simple splinters. Just make sure you gather it in a clean area where there is no traffic or animal pollution.

Fresh Comfrey Poultice

Comfrey is one of the most important plants to grow indoors as a first aid source. There are many stories which attest to the healing power of this plant, the principle ingredient of which, allantoin, is a cell proliferative. It is most useful as an external poultice to heal burns, stings, wounds and muscular sprains. Comfrey has traditionally been used to heal bone fractures.

Because it contains some potentially toxic alkaloids, it is best to take it internally only under the guidance of a competent herbalist or wholistic practitioner.

Ingredients:	Fresh Comfrey leaves
	Distilled water
Equipment:	Blender or mortar and pestle
	Gauze diaper (the thin Birds-eye kind)
	Roll gauze

Procedure: Pick the Comfrey leaves, rinse and shake them dry, then blend with enough distilled water to create a thick mash. Place in a gauze diaper, and apply to the treatment area, wrapping it with roll gauze to hold it in place. Occasionally you will see a skin rash developing due to small hairs that are found on the leaves. I have seen this in instances where the comfrey was applied directly to the skin. The gauze diaper should prevent this, however if the irritation persists, discontinue use, or, if it is not an open wound, smear a little olive oil on the area to be treated first. (If you need to, a poultice can also be made from the Comfrey root powder in the burn kit, see Dr. Christopher's burn ointment.)

Clay Poultice

Clay has been used to draw out toxins and foreign substances, heal burns and repair damaged tissue. Its virtues are endless and deserve study. In the beginning, start out with a simple green clay and observe the effects of the poultice.

Ingredients: 1 lb. pure green clay (Cattier is a good brand)
Distilled water (set 1/2 cup of clay powder aside for the face mask)

Equipment: Deep non-metal bowl
Wooden spoon
Diaper
Cotton gauze
Measuring cup
Sponge and towel

Procedure: Mix the clay with enough water to make a thick paste, spread with the spoon onto center of a thin gauze diaper or handkerchief in an area approximately 6" x 8" and 1" thick. Apply the clay directly to the part of the body to be treated, pressing it into the flesh so that it adheres. Cover with a dry cloth and leave it on until the clay pulls away on its own accord, indicating that the therapy is completed. For more information on clays, please read *The Healing Clay* by Michel Abehsera.

Onion Poultice

This poultice is used in cases of deep lung congestion and bronchial inflammation. It brings penetrating relief to that annoying itch of the lungs when it hurts too much to cough. It is also used over the ear and lymph glands to treat ear infections.

Ingredients: 3 large fresh onions (organically grown
                    if possible)
                 Distilled water

Equipment: Large glass or cast iron skillet
                 2 diapers or small towels
                 2 large towels
                 Rubber gloves
                 Wooden spoon or tongs

Procedure: Slice onions thinly and sauté them, covered, in a small amount of distilled water until transparent. Fold half of onions into a diaper so the finished pack is approximately 8" x 8". Apply to the chest as hot as the patient can stand it and immediately cover it with the towels to retain the heat. Begin preparing the next poultice. When the first one is cool, immediately replace it with the 2nd. After the therapy, gently dry the chest and tuck the patient into bed to rest. Use the same procedure for the ear, except make the poultice smaller.

Aloe Vera

This is one of the most useful first aid plants to grow indoors. Simply peel the outer structure of the leaf away to expose the inner gel, and wipe on minor burns, sunburns, cuts, scrapes, etc. You can also cut the inner gel into a suppository sized pellet and insert into the rectum as a hemorrhoid suppository.

Dr. Christopher's Burn Ointment

This formula has healed thousands of burns, and is unique in that it is not removed from the site of the injury, but is left on until the skin is completely healed. The Wheat Germ oil, Comfrey root, and Honey literally "feed" the tissue, soothing and promoting cell regeneration. It must be made fresh at the time it is needed, as it does not store well (turns into a blob of hard black goo). I highly recommend that you keep this in your medicine kit—just store the Wheat Germ oil and Honey in one container, and the Comfrey powder in another, then mix as needed.

Procedure: Stir equal parts Comfrey root powder, Wheat Germ oil and Honey together and apply liberally to the burn. Wrap in gauze to hold it on, replenish as necessary. Carry on with the treatment until the burn is completely healed and it will prevent scarring. If you get tired of wearing a bandage, you can start putting Wheat Germ or vitamin E alone on the burn after most of the healing work has been accomplished by the ointment. This period is identified by absence of pain and general tissue healing to the point that the skin has reformed and closed with a scab or pinkish red skin. Keep applying the oil on a daily basis until you cannot identify where the burn was.

Banana Peel Poultice for Warts

This therapy is easy. Look for brown-black bananas, the kind the grocer sells for 25 cents a pound. Take a section of the peel and place the inside part on the wart. Bind with roll gauze and leave on overnight, removing in the morning and replacing each night until the wart is gone.

Removing Moles

This therapy is not herbal, but it works so well I had to include it. I learned this method of removing moles from a macrobiotic cook, and have had 100% success with it. You first must be working with a mole that is protruding far enough to tie a hair around. Human hair works best, but *fine* unwaxed dental floss will also work. Simply tie the hair or floss into a circle and loop the end around an extra couple of times as if you are tieing shoes. This causes it to hold its position when you tighten it. Loop it carefully around the mole and pull it snugly, but not too tightly at first. Tighten each day until the mole drops off for lack of circulation.

Caution: If the mole is black or there is any other indication of abnormality, consult a qualified practitioner before commencing this therapy.

> **Fomentations:** Fomentations are either infusions or decoctions (depending on which part of the plant is used), in which a cloth is soaked to be applied to parts of the body needing therapy. Fomentations stimulate circulation, aid in decongestion, and can be soothing to external tissue.

Ginger Fomentation

This fomentation is especially good for cramps.

Ingredients: 1 cup fresh, grated Ginger root
2 quarts distilled water

Equipment: 4 quart saucepan
Cheesecloth
Rubber band
Thick diaper or cloth towels
Large bath towels

Procedure: Place Ginger root into cheesecloth, gather into a loose pouch and secure with a rubber band. Put the bag into the water and bring mixture to a boil, then reduce to a simmer. Simmer for 15 minutes (covered), remove from heat and strain. Carry the hot strained tea in a covered vessel to the patient's side. Dip a thick cloth such as a diaper into the tea. (Wearing plastic gloves will help.) Wring the cloth out and fan it in the air until it can be tested on the inside of your arm without scalding. It should be applied as hot as the patient can stand it, then covered with two towels to retain the heat as long as possible. After the cloth has cooled, remove and re-soak, then re-apply as before. Remember to keep the vessel covered between dippings to keep the liquid hot.

Decongesting Heat Lamp Therapy

This simple therapy is incredibly effective for sinuses that are so stuffed that you can't breathe through your nose at all and can't sleep. Just get an ordinary aluminum mechanic's light with a spring clip which is commonly available in most department stores. Install a heat lamp bulb in it. Clip it above you so that it can shine down on your sinuses. Cover your eyes, turn it on, and let the heat penetrate and decongest the area. Ahhhhh.

Cold Compress: This preparation is useful in preventing swelling and reducing fevers. It stimulates the production of both white and red blood cells and reduces the pulse rate. A decoction or infusion is prepared, allowed to cool and applied with a cloth as in the fomentation above.

Peppermint Cooling Compress

Ingredients: 1/2 cup Peppermint leaves
                    1 quart distilled water
                    Ice cubes

Equipment: 1 quart saucepan
                    Measuring cup
                    Thick diaper or cloth
                    Towel

Procedure: Pour boiling water over Peppermint leaves, cover and let steep for 10 minutes, strain and cool. When tea is lukewarm put it in the freezer or add ice cubes to make it really cold, then take to the patient. Soak a cloth in the tea and apply to the patient. The cloth should be wrung out so that it does not drip yet still retains enough liquid to stay cold. If the cloth warms up, re-soak and re-apply. Repeat this procedure three to five times, adding ice cubes if necessary, then dry the area thoroughly.

> **Vapors and Steams:** These preparations are useful for decongesting the lungs and detoxifying the skin. A vapor is prepared by dropping essential oils into freshly boiled distilled water, and a steam is essentially an infusion with the herbs left in it.

Decongestant Vapor

Ingredients: Muscle Ease salve formula or Eucalyptus oil
                   1 quart distilled water

Equipment: 4 quart glass or enamel pot
                   Towels
                   Headband

Procedure: Boil water, remove from heat, take a toothpick and scrape out a bit of Muscle salve (try a little at first, you can always add more), stir into the pan of water. Breathe in vapor while covering head with a towel to trap steam. (CAUTION: Steam burns are exceedingly unpleasant, so test the heat of the steam carefully with your hand before exposing your face.)

Cleansing Facial Steam

Ingredients: Lavender, Rosebud, and Chamomile flowers
                   (1/2 cup of mixture)
                   1 quart distilled water

Equipment: 4 quart glass or enamel pot
                   Towels
                   Headband

Procedure: Boil water, remove from heat, add herbs, stir into the pan of water. Let your face bathe in the vapor while covering head with a towel to trap steam. (See caution above.)

Herbal Eyewash

This eyewash is for tired, strained or infected eyes. It cleanses the tear ducts and stimulates circulation, which contributes to its fame as a vision restorative.

Ingredients: 1 tablespoon herb mixture: Eyebright, Red
                    Raspberry, Fennel, Goldenseal, Bayberry.
                1 cup distilled water

Equipment: 1 quart saucepan
                Eyecup
                Filter
                White paper towels or straining cloth
                2 bowls
                Ladle

Procedure: Boil water, take vessel from stove, add one tablespoon herb mix, let steep (covered), for 10 minutes. While the eyewash is steeping, sterilize the eyecup by boiling. Strain tea through a filter, cool till lukewarm. At this time the strained tea should be poured into a cup measure with a pour spout so that you can keep the batch sterile as you fill the eyecup (as opposed to dipping the eyecup in the solution to fill it). Fill the eye cup with the cooled solution, look down as you place it on your eye, then tip your head back, letting the solution wash the eye as you blink several times. It is helpful to hold a folded paper towel under the eye as you do this, to catch drips. Pour used solution into separate container and refill eyecup. Apply to same eye three separate times, then re-sterilize eyecup (this will prevent contamination of second eye) and repeat procedure on other eye. Eyewash should be made fresh each treatment as it does not store well in the refrigerator.

Castor Oil Pack

This is a remedy popularized by the late Edgar Cayce, and has proved very useful in stimulating deep tissue and organ healing. It has drawing power up to 4" deep in the tissue, and is used for deep infection, congestion and old, hard-to-heal injuries.

Ingredients:
- 6 ounces castor oil
- 1 teaspoon baking soda dissolved into:
- 1 pint cool water

Equipment:
- Wool flannel cloth
- Plastic sheet (a trash bag will do)
- Hot water bottle or electric heating pad
- Large bath towel

Procedure: Warm the castor oil by placing the bottle in a pan of hot water. Fold the flannel so that it is 4 layers thick with a surface area of approximately 10" x 14". Lay it on the plastic sheet and pour on the warmed oil so that it is thoroughly saturated but not dripping. Apply flannel to the area to be treated and cover with the plastic sheet, then place the heating source on top. If using the heating pad, turn it to medium then increase it to high if the patient can tolerate it. Leave it on for 1-8 hours. If using the hot water bottle, fill it 3/4 full, (not totally full or it won't curve around the body), place over sheet, and cover with a towel. Change water periodically to keep hot.

When the therapy is complete, remove the pack and cleanse the skin with the mixture of baking soda and water. Store the wool flannel in a plastic bag or glass jar in the refrigerator for further use. If it is not stored in the refrigerator it can go rancid.

THE HERBAL FIRST AID KIT

The following items are useful in the first aid kit and home medicine chest.

Aloe Burn Spray Formula
Antiseptic Spray Formula
Bug Spray Formula
Cramp Formula
Dental Poultices
Digestive Formula
Dr. Christopher's Burn Ointment
Herbal Eyewash kit (herbs, filter, eyecup)
Infection Formula
Itch Spray Formula
Laxative Formula
Mullein/Garlic Ear Oil Formula
Muscle/Bruise Salve or Liniment Spray Formula
Pain Formula
Restful Sleep Formula
Skin Soothing Salve Formula
Slippery Elm lozenges
Tea Tree Oil
Throat Extract/Spray Formula

Adhesive tape; bandages; cotton gauze, roll and pads (non-stick); eyecup; mirror; Q-Tips; scissors; thermometer (Oral and Rectal); tweezers

Other useful items: Castor Oil and wool flannel, cotton diapers, enema/douche bag, handkerchiefs, hot water bottle, large enamel or glass pot, First Aid Booklet or chart describing CPR and the Heimlich maneuver.

Materia Medica

A condensed, concise list of useful herbs and their therapeutic application. The pocket reference nature of this book makes it impossible to discuss everything the following herbs can be used for. The purpose is to get you started and to whet your appetite for more.

[P/C] indicates that the herb should be used with professional supervision and caution during pregnancy.

ALFALFA (Medicago sativa)
Nutritive herb with high mineral and vitamin content including Vit. K and iron; estrogen precursor for menopause; mild diuretic.

ALOE (Aloe vera) [P/C]
Applied fresh as a burn and wound remedy, astringent. Fresh peeled leaf gel inserted as a rectal suppository for hemorrhoids. For chronic constipation with atonic bowel.

ANGELICA ROOT (Angelica spp.) [P/C]
Antispasmodic, for strong menstrual cramps with scanty flow; intestinal colic and poor digestion; stimulating expectorant for coughs.

ANISE SEED (Pimpinella anisum)
Eases indigestion, flatulence and colic. Antispasmodic and expectorant.

ARNICA FLOWER (Arnica cordifolia) [External Use Only]
Topical use for bruises, sprains, strains and other athletic injuries, including swelling. Use on unbroken skin.

BALM OF GILEAD (Populus balsamifera)
Soothes, disinfects and astringes mucous membranes. Specific for laryngitis, coughs and sore throat.

BARBERRY ROOT (Berberis fendleri) [P/C]
Digestive and appetite stimulant; stimulates bile flow and liver function; refrigerant; reduces fevers; antiseptic. Anticonvulsant.

BAYBERRY BARK (Myrica cerifera)
Astringent, used for bleeding gums and sore throat, diarrhea, gastrointestinal inflammation, post partum hemorrhage; vasodilator of skin and mucus membranes.

BETH ROOT (Trillium erectum) [P/C]
Uterine tonic containing natural precursor of female sex hormones. Astringent, used for excess menstrual flow, postpartum hemorrhage.

BILBERRY (Vaccinum myrtillus)
Astringent, antiseptic, absorptive, anti-emetic. Used for intestinal dyspepsia and to halt diarrhea. Helps heal irritated intestinal mucosa resulting from chronic constipation. Large quantities of freshly ripened berries, eaten raw, are laxative. Used as anti-inflammatory mouthwash. Used to enhance vision when taken for long periods of time.

BISTORT (Polygonum bistorta)
Astringent; anti-inflammatory; used for diarrhea, dysentery, mouth inflammations, laryngitis, pharyngitis.

BLACK COHOSH ROOT (Cimicifuga racemosa) [P/C]
Antispasmodic used for menstrual cramping, coughs, muscle spasms; emmenagogue; relieves hot flashes in menopausal women; mild sedative.

BLACK WALNUT HULLS (Juglans nigra)
Antifungal, (for Candida, athlete's foot, ringworm, etc.); astringent, used for skin eruptions; vermifuge in larger doses. Helps break down cystic tissue.

BLADDERWRACK (Fucus vesiculosus)
Thyroid balancer, specific in treating obesity associated with under-active thyroid. Anti-rheumatic. Alleviates diarrhea and hemorrhage.

BLESSED THISTLE (Cnicus benedictus)
Increases lactation; emmenagogue; carminative, for indigestion and chronic headaches; astringent, for diarrhea and hemorrhage.

BLOODROOT (Sanguinaria canadensis)
Expectorant. For chronic bronchitis, croup, laryngitis. Gargle for mouth sores and plaque build up. Topical for eczema.

BLUE COHOSH (Caulophyllum thalictroides) [P/C]
Uterine tonic, emmenagogue; diuretic; Antispasmodic; diaphoretic; mild expectorant. Helps prevent threatened miscarriage. *For use in last trimester only.*

BLUE FLAG ROOT (Iris versicolor)
Liver purgative; blood purifier; cathartic; sialagogue; diuretic. For constipation and biliousness, eruptive skin conditions. *Low doses only.*

BLUE VERVAIN (Verbena spp.)
Soothes cranky children, sedative, anti-depressant, diaphoretic, febrifuge, antispasmodic, mild analgesic.

BONESET (Eupatorium perfoliatum)
For flu symptoms, aches and pains; clears mucus congestion; reduces fevers; muscular rheumatism.

BORAGE LEAF (Borago officinalis)
Restorative for adrenal cortex, especially after cortisone or steroid treatment. Diaphoretic; expectorant; anti-inflammatory; anti-depressant; galactagogue.

BUCKTHORN BARK (Rhamnus frangula)
Moderately strong laxative, very useful in chronic constipation. Must be dried before use to avoid intestinal cramping and nausea.

BURDOCK ROOT (Arctium lappa)
Blood cleanser, anti-microbial. Used for skin eruptions, dry/scaly skin conditions; digestive stimulant. Lowers blood sugar. Cancer preventative.

BURDOCK SEED (Arctium lappa)
Diuretic, kidney tonic, demulcent. Specific for chronic skin disease.

BUTTERBUR (Petasites hybridus)
Muscle relaxant, used for intestinal colic, asthma, painful menses; mild febrifuge.

BUTTERNUT BARK (Juglans cinerea)
Mild laxative; hepatic decongestant; vermifuge. Used for dysentery.

CALENDULA FLOWER (Calendula officinalis)

Anti-inflammatory; astringent; styptic; antifungal; emmenagogue; cholagogue; topically for wounds, ulcers, burns, abscesses.

CASCARA SAGRADA BARK (Rhamnus purshiana) [P/C]

Laxative, mild liver stimulant, bitter tonic.

CATNIP HERB (Nepeta cataria)

Carminative, diaphoretic, antispasmodic, mild febrifuge. For indigestion, flatulence and colic; mild astringent, specific for childhood fevers and diarrhea.

CAYENNE FRUIT (Capsicum frutescens)

Equalizes circulation, for cold hands and feet; strengthens heart; stimulant; carminative; styptic. Antiseptic, used as gargle for persistent cough.

CHAMOMILE FLOWER (Matricaria recutita)

Sedative, carminative, antispasmodic, anodyne. Children's herb, especially for fever and restlessness. Mouthwash for gingivitis.

CHAPARRAL LEAF (Larrea tridentata)

Blood cleanser, antioxidant; antibiotic; anti-viral; antiseptic; specific for infections, sluggish liver, skin problems, arthritis, tumors.

CHAPARRO (Castela emoryi)

Active inhibitor of intestinal protozoa. Used to prevent and alleviate amoebic dysentery and giardia.

CHASTE BERRY (Vitex agnus castus)

Reproductive tonic, stimulates and normalizes pituitary function. For menstrual cramps, PMS, menopause, post birth control pill rebalancing.

CHICKWEED HERB (Stellaria media)
Nutritive; restorative; demulcent; diuretic; regulates thyroid; high in saponins, (increases cell membrane permeability) and lecithin, (emulsifies and mobilizes fat).

CLEAVERS (Galium spp.)
Lymphatic tonic; alterative; diuretic. For swollen glands, cystitis, ulcers and tumors, skin disorders, painful urination.

COLTSFOOT (Tussilago farfara)
Soothing expectorant, demulcent, antispasmodic, astringent, anti-inflammatory. For irritating coughs, bronchitis, asthma, laryngitis, throat catarrh; externally for sores and ulcers.

COMFREY ROOT/LEAF (Symphytum officinalis)
Speeds healing of sprains, strains, fractures and surface wounds. *Is not currently recommended for internal use.*

CORIANDER SEED (Coriandrum sativum)
Carminative, eases intestinal griping and diarrhea (especially in children). Appetite stimulant, increases secretion of gastric juices.

CORN SILK (Zea mays)
Soothing diuretic, for renal and urinary irritation; used for bedwetting, cystitis, urethritis, prostatitis.

COTTON ROOT (Gossypium herbaceum)
Works in conjunction with oxytocin to increase contractibility of uterus, seminal vesicles, and mammary tissue. Aids ability to ejaculate. Helps stimulate post-partum contractions. Useful to aid withdrawal from birth control pills.

COUCHGRASS ROOT (Agropyron repens)
Demulcent; anti-microbial; antilithic; for cystitis, urethritis, prostatitis, kidney stones and gravel.

COW PARSNIP ROOT/SEED (Heracleum lanatum)
Anti-nauseant; stimulant; hypotensive; emmenagogue; antispasmodic; carminative. Analgesic for sore teeth and gums.

CRAMP BARK (Viburnum opulus)
Relaxes muscle tension and spasms, ovarian and uterine cramps. Used to prevent threatened miscarriage.

CRANBERRY (Vaccinium oxycoccus)
Diuretic and urinary antiseptic; for kidney and bladder infections.

DAMIANA (Turnera diffusa)
Diuretic, relieves irritation of urinary mucus membranes; genito-urinary stimulant effect leading to its use as an aphrodisiac; improves digestion; laxative; tonic; relieves bronchial irritation and coughs.

DANDELION ROOT/LEAF (Taraxacum officinale)
Blood cleanser; powerful and safe diuretic, high in potassium; cholagogue, for inflammation and congestion of the liver and gall bladder, congestive jaundice. Mild laxative, aids weight loss, lowers cholesterol and blood pressure.

DESERT WILLOW LEAF/BARK (Chilopsis linearis)
Anti-fungal. Used to treat Candida albicans, specifically the symptoms of candida suprainfections which are abundant after antibiotic therapy, i.e. indigestion, loose stools, hemorrhoids, rectal aching, foul burping, etc.

DEVIL'S CLUB (Oplopanax horridus)
Pancreatic tonic, blood sugar regulator, increases endurance.

DILL SEED (Anethum graveolens)
For flatulence and colic, especially in children; stimulates lactation.

DONG QUAI ROOT (Angelica sinensis)
Female hormone regulator, alleviates cramping and premenstrual distress.

ECHINACEA ROOT (Echinacea angustifolia)
Powerful immune stimulant; antiseptic; anti-microbial; antiviral; used for sore throats, flu, colds, infections, allergies.

ELDER FLOWERS (Sambucus canadensis)
Diaphoretic, anti-catarrhal, diuretic, expectorant. For upper respiratory infections, colds, flu, hayfever, sinusitis, fevers.

ELECAMPANE ROOT (Inula helenium)
Expectorant; diaphoretic; anti-bacterial; anti-tussive; stomachic; for irritating bronchial coughs, bronchitis, emphysema, asthma and bronchitic asthma.

EPHEDRA (Ephedra spp.) *Mormon Tea*
Vasodilator; antispasmodic; hypertensive; circulatory stimulant; used for asthma, bronchitis, whooping cough, hayfever; opens air passages.

EYEBRIGHT HERB (Euphrasia officinalis)
Anti-catarrhal, astringent, anti-inflammatory. Internally for sinusitis, nasal congestion, eye inflammations. Used as an external infusion/wash for sore or inflamed eyes.

FALSE UNICORN (Helonias) (Chamaelirium luteum)
Uterine tonic, used for delayed menses, leukorrhea, ovarian pain. Contains estrogen precursors. Eases vomiting in pregnancy (small doses). Helps prevent threatened miscarriage.

FENNEL SEED (Foeniculum vulgare)
Aids digestion; relieves flatulence and colic; expels mucus; increases lactation; aids weight loss; flavoring agent; increases digestibility of other herbs.

FENUGREEK SEED (Trigonella-foenum-graecum)
Soothes irritated mucus membranes, promotes lactation, mild febrifuge.

FEVERFEW LEAF/FLOWER (Tanacetum parthenium)
Anti-inflammatory, used for rheumatoid arthritis, migraine headache relief (long term basis), asthma and bronchitis. Mild febrifuge, especially good for children. Used topically to relieve swelling from insect bites.

FIGWORT HERB (Scrophularia spp.)
Used internally and topically for eczema, scrofula, cradle cap, psoriasis, itching and irritated skin. *Avoid in cases of tachycardia.*

FLAX SEED (Linum usitatissimum)
Excellent bulking agent which cleanses and lubricates digestive tract.

FRINGETREE BARK (Chionanthus virginicus)
Hepatic; cholagogue; alterative; diuretic. Used for liver problems, gall bladder inflammation and stones. Gentle, effective laxative.

GARLIC BULB/SEED (Alliumsativum)

Antibiotic; anti-microbial; antiseptic; antiviral; anthelmintic. For colds, flu, chronic bronchitis, infections, also to reduce blood pressure and cholesterol.

GENTIAN ROOT (Gentiana lutea)

Bitter, promotes production of gastric juices and bile. For sluggish digestion, dyspepsia and flatulence. Restores appetite lost during morning sickness.

GINGER ROOT (Zinziber officinalis)

Used for nausea, motion sickness; diaphoretic, helps break fevers; stimulant; carminative; aids in utilization of other herbs.

GINKGO LEAF (Ginkgo biloba)

Stimulates cerebral circulation and oxygenation, mental clarity and alertness, improves memory. Used to prevent strokes.

GINSENG ROOT (Panax quinquefolium)

Adaptogenic, decreases the effect of stress. Increases capillary circulation in brain; reproductive tonic; anti-depressant; equalizes blood pressure. Used for general exhaustion and weakness; aids digestion. Promotes longevity.

GOLDENROD (Solidago virgauria)

Anti-inflammatory; urinary antiseptic; diuretic; diaphoretic; expectorant, astringent. For cystitis, urethritis, upper respiratory catarrh, diarrhea and internal hemorrhage. Gargle for laryngitis and pharyngitis. Diaphoretic, sedative, carminative. Reduces congestion.

GOLDENSEAL ROOT (Hydrastis canadensis)

Antiseptic, used for internally and topically for infection, sore throat, gastritis ulceration and colitis. Root infusion used as douche for vaginitis. Should not be taken daily for more than a week or so as overuse can stress the liver.

GOTU KOLA LEAF (Centella asiatica)
Used to increase mental stamina, alleviate depression and anxiety, improve memory and promote longevity. Increases energy and endurance.

GRAVEL ROOT (Eupatorium purpureum)
For kidney and urinary infections and stones, prostatitis, pelvic inflammatory disease; painful menses; rheumatism and gout.

GRINDELIA BUDS/FLOWERS (Grindelia spp.)
Expectorant; anti-spasmodic; for bronchitis, sinus congestion, bladder infections; topically for poison oak and ivy, insect bites.

HAWTHORNE BERRY (Crataegus oxycantha)
Heart and circulatory tonic. Used for heart weakness, palpitations, high blood pressure, arteriosclerosis, angina pectoris.

HOPS STROBILE (Humulus lupulus)
Sedative; hypnotic. Used for anxiety, tension, insomnia. Reduces nervous irritability, promotes restful sleep. Astringent, used for mucous colitis.

HOREHOUND HERB (Marrubium vulgare)
Excellent expectorant for respiratory congestion.

HORSERADISH ROOT (Armoracia rusticana)
Stimulant; for flu, fevers, sinus and respiratory congestion. Sialagogue, carminative, mild laxative, diuretic.

HORSETAIL HERB (Equisetum arvense)
High in silica and calcium, used to strengthen hair, skin and nails.

HYDRANGEA ROOT (Hydrangea aborescens)
Diuretic, cathartic, tonic. Helps evacuate gravelly deposits from the bladder and alleviates the pain of their passage. Styptic. Helps correct bedwetting in children.

HYSSOP LEAF (Hyssopus officinalis)
Anti-spasmodic; nervine; expectorant; diaphoretic, sedative, carminative. For chronic congestion.

INMORTAL ROOT (Asclepius asperula)
Bronchial dilator; stimulates lymph drainage from the lungs. Used for asthma, pleurisy, bronchitis, lung infections. Laxative, diaphoretic, mild cardiac tonic.

JEWELWEED (Impatiens aurens) External Use
Used topically to reduce the itching and inflammation of skin irritating plants such as poison ivy.

JUNIPER BERRY (Juniperus spp.)
Urinary tract antiseptic, used for cystitis, urethritis. Should not be used in kidney inflammation or chronic kidney weakness.

JAMAICAN DOGWOOD (Piscidia erythrina)
Sedative; anodyne; smooth muscle antispasmodic. For insomnia, neuralgia, menstrual cramping. Relieves coughing, reduces fevers.

KELP (Nereocystis luetkeana)
Radiation protective properties. Reduces amount of strontium-90 absorbed by bone tissue by 50-85%

LEMON BALM (Melissa officinalis)
Very useful in reducing fevers during colds and flu as it induces mild perspiration. Aids digestion, reduces flatulence.

Wonderful herb for children. Anti-viral, used externally on herpes lesions.

LICORICE ROOT (Glycyrrhiza glabra)
Specific for adrenal gland insufficiency; demulcent; expectorant for coughs and respiratory congestion; anti-inflammatory; laxative.

LOBELIA HERB (Lobelia inflata)
Respiratory stimulant; anti-asthmatic; anti-emetic (small dose), emetic (large dose); used for bronchitis and bronchitic asthma, whooping cough, muscular cramping and pain.

LOMATIUM ROOT (Lomatium dissectum)
Antiviral; immune stimulant; for colds, flu, viral sore throats, respiratory infections and congestion.

MARSHMALLOW ROOT (Althaea officinalis)
Soothing demulcent, used for gastrointestinal inflammation; expectorant in respiratory congestion and bronchitis. Used externally as a poultice for mastitis and skin ulcers.

MEADOWSWEET (Filipendula ulmaria)
Digestive herb, antacid. Used for heartburn, nausea, gastritis, hyperacidity, peptic ulcers. Mild astringent, used for diarrhea in children. Diaphoretic, anti-inflammatory, reduces fever and pain.

MILK THISTLE SEED (Silybum marianum)
Powerful liver detoxifier, antidote for Amanita mushroom poisoning. Increases secretion and flow of bile. Galactagogue.

MOTHERWORT HERB (Leonurus cardiaca) [P/C]

Sedative, useful in transition labor. Eases false labor pains. Antispasmodic; emmenagogue; cardiac tonic; reduces tension, anxiety.

MULLEIN LEAF (Verbascum thapsus)

Expectorant; demulcent; reduces respiratory inflammation. Flowers steeped in olive oil used as an earache remedy.

MYRRH GUM (Commiphora myrrha)

Antiseptic; anti-microbial; astringent. Used for mouth ulcers, sore throat, gingivitis, pyorrhea, sinusitis and pharyngitis. Used externally on cuts and abrasions, forms natural bandage.

NETTLE (Urtica dioica)

Nutritive herb, specific for childhood and nervous eczema. Rich in iron, silica, and potassium. For anemia. Diuretic; galactagogue; antihistamine; for hayfever and allergies.

OATSEED (Avena sativa)

Antispasmodic; soothes and supports nervous system; for depression, insomnia, hysteria, irritation and anxiety. Helpful in breaking addictions.

OCOTILLO (Fouquieria splendens)

Stimulates lymphatic drainage; improves dietary fat absorption into the lymph system. Helps drain pelvic congestion, making it useful in the treatment of hemorrhoids and varicose veins.

ONION (Allium cepa)

Diuretic, expectorant, carminative, antiseptic, antispasmodic, anthelmintic. Helps alleviate putrefaction in the gastrointestinal tract. Used to alleviate cold and flu symptoms.

OREGON GRAPE ROOT (Mahonia repens)
Liver and blood cleanser; cholagogue; anti-bacterial. Stimulates digestion and absorption. For sluggish liver, hangovers, acne, eczema.

OSHA' ROOT (Ligusticum porterii)
Strong antiviral, used for herpes, sore throat, colds, flu; bronchial expectorant; immune stimulating properties.

PARSLEY LEAF / ROOT (Petroselenum crispum) [P/C]
Diuretic, carminative, antispasmodic, emmenagogue, expectorant.

PASSIONFLOWER (Passiflora incarnata)
Sedative, hypnotic, antispasmodic, anodyne. Relieves nerve pain, promotes restful sleep. Has been used for seizures and hysteria.

PAU D' ARCO (Tabebuia impetiginosa)
Blood cleanser; anti-fungal; for candida, lymph congestion, tumors. Improves gastrointestinal utilization of nutrients.

PEPPERMINT LEAF (Mentha piperita)
For upset stomach, heartburn, nausea, colds, flu, congestion, nervous headache and agitation, also diarrhea and flatulence. Adds flavor to other herbs.

PIPSISSEWA (Chimaphila umbellata)
Diuretic, used for chronic kidney weakness, nephritis, bladder stones and rheumatism.

PLANTAIN LEAF (Plantago spp.)
Expectorant; astringent; for coughs, bronchitis, diarrhea, hemorrhoids, bleeding cystitis, chronic catarrhal problems, external wounds and sores, insect bites, hoarseness, gastritis.

PLEURISY ROOT (Asclepias tuberosa)

Respiratory infections, bronchitis, pleurisy, pneumonia, flu. Reduces inflammation and encourages expectoration.

POKE ROOT (Phytolacca americana)

Emetic, purgative. Cleanses lymph, for tonsillitis, mumps, laryngitis, swollen glands mastitis, rheumatism. Small doses only. *Physician or Herbalist supervision advised.*

POTENTILLA (Potentilla spp.)

Astringent mouthwash and gargle for sore throats or gum inflammation. Used for stomach ulcers, abrasions, sunburn, poison oak, fevers, diarrhea.

PROPOLIS

Antiseptic, antibacterial. Waxy nature makes it useful for coating and isolating areas of throat inflammation to prevent spread of infection.

PSYLLIUM SEED (Plantago ovata)

Commonly called the intestinal janitor, softly "scrubs" the sides of the intestinal wall for maximum cleansing effect.

QUASSIA (Pycrasma excelsa)

Bitter tonic and stomachic; antispasmodic; anthelmintic. Used to rid the body of parasites and improve digestion.

RED CLOVER FLOWERS (Trifolium pratense)

Blood cleanser; nutritive; for childhood eczema, psoriasis, coughs, bronchitis, ulcers, inflammation and infection. Galactagogue. Principal ingredient of the Hoxey cancer formula.

RED RASPBERRY LEAF (Rhubus idaeus)

Pregnancy herb; nutritive; relieves nausea. Uterine tonic, eases painful menses, checks hemorrhage. Remedy for childhood diarrhea, gargle for sore throat, bleeding gums.

RED ROOT (Ceanothus americanus)

Stimulates lymphatic and interstitial fluid circulation, aids in the transport of nutrients and the elimination of waste products. Used for tonsillitis, sore throat, enlarged lymph nodes and spleen, fibrous cysts. Expectorant, hemostatic.

REISHI MUSHROOM (Ganoderma lucidum)

Adaptogenic, used to alleviate the effects of stress. Strengthens heart, protects liver, soothes nerves. Normalizes blood pressure. Inhibits the release of histamine, thus relieving the allergic inflammatory response. Supports adrenal function. Stimulates the immune system. Slows the aging process. Anti-carcinogenic.

RHUBARB ROOT (Rheum officinale) [P/C]

Stomachic, astringent, small doses relieve diarrhea, large doses laxative.

ROSEHIPS (Rosa canina)

Nutrient, mild diuretic and laxative, mild astringent. Excellent source of vitamin C. Used for colds, flu, general debility and exhaustion, constipation.

ROSEMARY LEAF (Rosmarinus officinalis)

Circulatory and nerve stimulant, used for tension headache associated with dyspepsia, also depression. Anti-bacterial; anti-fungal. Externally for muscular pain, neuralgia and sciatica.

SARSAPARILLA ROOT (Smilax ornata)
Anti-rheumatic, diuretic, diaphoretic, soothes mucous membranes, possible progesterone precursor.

SAW PALMETTO (Serenoa repens)
Tones and strengthens male reproductive system, used for prostate enlargement and infection, enhances endurance. Female fertility aid, galactagogue.

SHIITAKE MUSHROOM (Lentinus edodes)
Adaptogenic. Increases the production of interferon, thus reducing the possibility of tumor development. Anti-viral. Helps the body excrete excess cholesterol.

SHEPHERD'S PURSE (Capsella Bursa-pastoris)
Hemostatic; astringent; helps stop passive uterine or gastrointestinal bleeding. Diuretic; breaks up urinary stones.

SIBERIAN GINSENG (Eleutherococcus senticosis)
Stimulates the adrenal-pituitary axis, increasing resistance to stress. Improves cerebral circulation, increasing mental alertness.

SKULLCAP HERB (Scutellaria lateriflora)
Nervine; sedative; antispasmodic; used for nervous tension, hysteria, epileptic seizures, withdrawal from substance abuse and the irritability of PMS.

SLIPPERY ELM (Ulmus rubra)
Nutrient, reduces inflammation, soothes mucus membranes, specific for ulcers.

SPILANTHES (Spilanthes oleracea)
Anti-fungal, anti-bacterial; used for Candidiasis. Anodyne, anesthetic, relieves toothache.

SPIKENARD (Aralia racemosa)
Stimulant, diaphoretic, expectorant, alterative. Used for coughs and asthma.

SQUAWVINE/PARTRIDGE BERRY (Mitchella repens)
Uterine tonic, promotes easy labor, eases menstrual cramping, mild nervine, improves digestion.

STILLINGIA ROOT (Stillingia sylvatica)
Stimulating expectorant for bronchitis; blood cleanser, used for skin disorders. Small dose laxative and diuretic, large dose cathartic and emetic.

ST. JOHN'S WORT (Hypericum perforatum)
Extract and oil used externally for bruises, strains, sprains, contusions, wounds. Extract used internally as an immune system stimulant; for retro-viral infections; expectorant; antibacterial, speeds wound and burn healing; antidepressant; used to treat bedwetting and children's nightmares.

STONE ROOT (Collinsonia canadensis)
Strengthens structure and function of veins, used for varicose veins, hemorrhoids, anal fissures, and rectal spasms. Strong diuretic, helps prevent and dissolve urinary stones and gravel.

THYME LEAF (Thymus vulgaris)
Anti-bacterial; anti-fungal; anti-microbial; anti-spasmodic; expectorant; astringent, anthelmintic; diaphoretic. Used as throat gargle for laryngitis, tonsillitis, sore throats, coughs. Reduces fevers, expels worms.

TOADFLAX (Linaria vulgaris)
Liver cleanser; stimulates bile production; used in hepatitis, jaundice, sluggish liver. Potent—best used in small amounts in formulas.

TRONADORA (Tecoma stans)
Anti-viral, particularly helpful for herpes simplex, use internally.

USNEA LICHEN (Usnea spp.)
Strong antibiotic; antiviral; antifungal; for internal infections, strep, staph, trichomonas, etc., infected wounds. Also used for pneumonia, TB and Lupus.

UVA URSI (Arcostaphylos uva-ursi)
Urinary antiseptic; anti-microbial; for cystitis, urethritis, prostatitis, nephritis. Antilithic, used for kidney and bladder stones.

VALERIAN ROOT (Valeriana officinalis)
Powerful nervine, used for tension, anxiety, insomnia, emotional stress, intestinal colic, menstrual cramps, migraine headache and rheumatic pain.

WAHOO (Euonymus atropurpureus)
Primary liver decongestant, bile stimulant; used for jaundice, gall-bladder pain and inflammation, constipation.

WATERCRESS (Nasturtium officinalis)
Expectorant, diuretic, appetite stimulant, aids digestion.

WHITE OAK BARK (Quercus alba)
Astringent, used for diarrhea, hemorrhage, leucorrhea, bleeding or ulcerated gums. Topically for sores, hemorrhoids. Strengthens capillaries.

WHITE WILLOW BARK (Salix alba)
Astringent, contains salicin, reduces inflammation. Used for headache, neuralgia, fevers, hayfever, arthritis and rheumatism.

WILD CHERRY BARK (Prunus serotina)
Expectorant, anti-tussive, astringent, sedative, digestive bitter.
Used for irritating coughs, bronchitis and asthma.

WILD GERANIUM (Geranium maculatum)
Astringent, used for diarrhea and hemorrhage, bleeding gums,
hemorrhoids.

WILD GINGER (Asarum canadense)
Diaphoretic, expectorant, carminative. Relieves flatulence, colic
and upset stomach. Expels mucus. Helps reduce fevers by causing mild sweating, thus dropping the body temperature. Not as
hot as the cultivated Ginger (Zinziber officinalis).

WILD INDIGO ROOT (Baptisia tinctoria)
Emetic; purgative; lymph cleanser; for focused local infection
such as sore throat, laryngitis, tonsillitis, pharyngitis, gingivitis,
mouth ulcers and pyorrhea. Also inflamed lymph nodes. Best
used in small amounts in a formula. *Caution: Large doses may be
toxic.*

WILD LETTUCE HERB (Lactuca spp.)
Sedative, calms restlessness and anxiety, subdues irritating
coughs.

WILD YAM ROOT (Dioscorea spp.)
Antispasmodic; carminative; anti-inflammatory; hepatic;
cholagogue; diaphoretic. Used for intestinal colic, diverticulitis,
painful menses, ovarian and uterine pain, rheumatoid arthritis,
flatulence.

WORMWOOD LEAF (Artemisia absinthium)
Brings down fevers: will inhibit roundworm and pinworm infestation when used consistently for a week or two. Stimulates

sweating in dry fevers. Aids uterine circulation. *Use small amounts, preferably with herbalist or physician supervision.*

YARROW FLOWERS (Achillea millefolium)
Diaphoretic, helps release toxic waste and reduce fevers. Lowers blood pressure; specific for thrombotic conditions associated with high blood pressure.

YELLOW DOCK ROOT (Rumex crispus)
Blood cleanser, used for anemia, hepatitis, chronic skin disorders. Mild laxative, aids fat digestion.

YERBA MANSA ROOT (Anemopsis californica)
Soothing to mucus membranes, used for diarrhea, dysentery, malarial fevers, gonorrhea, catarrh, digestive weakness.

YERBA SANTA LEAF (Eriodycton spp.)
Expectorant; bronchial dilator; mild decongestant, for chest colds, asthma, hayfever, bronchitis.

YUCCA ROOT (Yucca spp.)
Anti-inflammatory, used for arthritic pain, rheumatism, gout, asthma, urethral and prostate inflammation.

Dosages, Weights and Measures

DOSAGES

Always a sticky subject due to personal metabolism, dietary habits, stress levels and other vagaries of our individual bodies, dosage guidelines are nevertheless important. Well put in Felter's *Materia Medica*, Vol. 1, "It is better to err on the side of insufficient dosage and trust to nature, than to overdose to the present or future harm or danger to the patient." In other words, try a little and watch for the patient's reaction before you give a lot. In my own body (and truly, this is my best teacher), I take a dropperful every hour if I am fighting off an acute infection, and usually take a dropperful per day in chronic problems. The dose also depends on the potency of the preparation, so the variables are endless. If one is sensitive enough, and listens well to one's own body, the dosage should be apparent.

If you have any questions after researching the excellent sources in the book list, by all means see a competent wholistic practitioner who can help you figure it out. The following is a list of comparative children's dosages.

Cowling's rule: Divide the age at the next birthday by 24. (Example: A five year old child—six being the age at the next birthday—divide 6 by 24 which gives you 6/24 or 1/4 the adult dose.)

Clark's rule: Divide the weight (in lbs.) of the child by 150 to give the approximate fraction of the adult dose. (Example: A 50 lb. child will require 50/150 or 1/3 the adult dose.)

Young's rule: Computed by dividing the child's age by 12 plus the age. (Thus for a child of 4 years, it would be 4 divided by 12 + 4 = 4/16 = 1/4 of the adult dosage.)

WEIGHTS AND MEASURES

Liquid Equivalents (Volume)
1 oz. = 29.57 ml.
1 pt. = 16 oz. = 473.3 ml.
1 qt. = 2 pt. = 4 cups = 32 oz. = 946.6 ml.
1 Gal. = 4 Qts. = 8 Pts. = 16 cups = 128 oz. = 3,784.95 ml.

Solid Equivalents (Weight)
1 oz. = 28.4 gr.
1 lb. = 16 oz. = 453.6 gr.
1 kg. = 2.2 lb. = 35.2 oz. = 1,000 gr.

HERBAL EXTRACT MEASUREMENTS

The following information will be useful in dispensing herbal extracts and determining how long a bottle will last, depending on the dosage specified.

Rubber stoppers sometimes give the extract a rubbery taste, and some people prefer to use extracts which are not stored with the dropper. Therefore I am including the dosage measurements by the teaspoon as well as by drops or droppers full.

Accuracy of measurement is difficult when prescribing drops (minims). 20 drops of one extract may not equal the volume of a different extract due to glycerin content, sediment, manufacturer's design, etc. Water forms a larger droplet, while a droplet of single herbal extract is smaller. A combination extract which contains vegetable glycerin also changes the volume, as noted on the next page.

10 ml water = 265-297 drops, depending on speed of expulsion.
10 ml. single extract of Osha' Rt = 440 drops.
10 ml. combination extract = 447 drops.

Two ounce bottles have longer droppers and contain more fluid per filling than the one ounce dropper.

1 oz. size = approximately 30 drops per dropper.
2 oz. size = approximately 40 drops per dropper.

One Ounce Bottle (Single or combination extract):

- Holds *approximately* 29.57 ml. of fluid.
- 4 ml. = 1 teaspoonful
- 1 dropperful = *approximately* 1 ml. = *approx.* 1/4 teaspoon
- 1 oz. bottle holds *approximately* 7.4 teaspoons.
- Average 30-40 drops (minims) per glass dropper (1 oz. size)
- *Approximately* 29.5 droppersful per bottle
- *Approximately* 1,000-1,200 drops per bottle, depending on formula constituents.

- At a quantity of "One dropperful, three times daily," a one ounce bottle would last approximately 10 days.

- At a quantity of "Twenty drops, three times daily," a one ounce bottle would last approximately 18 days.

Recommended Reading List

I do not intend for this to be an herbal bibliography. There are many other fine books out there, but I have found these to be particularly useful to beginning students of herbal medicine. A more complete bibliography can be found in my video herbal reference manual. Enjoy.

Willard, Terry, *Helping Yourself with Natural Remedies*, CRCS, 1986

Nuzzi, Debra, *Herbal Preparations and Natural Therapies—Creating and Using a Home Herbal Medicine Chest*, Morningstar Publications, Boulder, CO, 1989. (303)444-7610

Thrash and Thrash, *Home Remedies*. Thrash Publications, Seale, AL, 1981

Rina Nissim, *Natural Healing in Gynecology*, Pandora Press, 1986

Santillo, Humbart, *Natural Healing With Herbs*, Hohm Press, 1984

Tierra, Michael, *Planetary Herbology*, Lotus Press, 1988

Wren, R.C., *Potter's New Cyclopedia of Botanical Drugs and Preparations*, Daniel, 1985

Lust, John, *The Herb Book*. Bantam, 1979

Tierra, Lesley, *The Herbs of Life*, The Crossing Press, 1992

Hoffman, David, *The Holistic Herbal*. Thornton, 1991

Vogel, H.C.A., *The Nature Doctor*, Mainstream Pub.,1990

Mabey, Richard, *The New Age Herbalist*. MacMillan, NY, 1988

Gardner, Joy, *The New Healing Yourself*. The Crossing Press, Freedom, CA, 1989

If you are pregnant and are concerned about herbs which should not be used during pregnancy, consult these books:

Gardner, Joy, *Healing the Family*, Bantam, 1982

Gardner, Joy, *Healing Yourself during Pregnancy*.The Crossing Press, 1987

Weed, Susan, *The WiseWoman Herbal for the Childbearing Year*. Ash Tree Pub. NY 1985

INDEX